GO WILD

EAT FAT, RUN FREE, BE SOCIAL, AND
FOLLOW EVOLUTION'S OTHER RULES FOR
TOTAL HEALTH AND WELL-BEING

JOHN J. RATEY, MD
and RICHARD MANNING

Foreword by David Perlmutter, MD

LITTLE, BROWN AND COMPANY
New York   Boston   London

Little, Brown and Company
Hachette Book Group
1290 Avenue of the Americas, New York, NY 10104
littlebrown.com

Originally published in hardcover by Little, Brown and Company, June 2014
First Little, Brown and Company trade paperback edition, December 2015

Little, Brown and Company is a division of Hachette Book Group, Inc. The Little, Brown name and logo are trademarks of Hachette Book Group, Inc.

The publisher is not responsible for websites (or their content) that are not owned by the publisher.

The Hachette Speakers Bureau provides a wide range of authors for speaking events. To find out more, go to hachettespeakersbureau.com or call (866) 376-6591.

The photograph on page 11 is reprinted with permission of Getty Images / Nat Farbman.

ISBN 978-0-316-24609-5 (hc) / 978-0-316-24610-1 (pb)
Library of Congress Control Number 2014936317

10 9 8 7 6 5 4 3

LSC-C

Printed in the United States of America

Contents

Foreword

On March 7, 2009, NASA launched the *Kepler* space observatory with the goal of discovering earthlike planets orbiting stars in our galaxy. Almost immediately, the data produced by this venture revealed the presence of planets orbiting stars in the "Goldilocks zone," a term used to describe an ideal distance between a planet and its parent star that is "neither too hot nor too cold"—what scientists have more formally termed the "habitable zone." By November 2013, the mission scientists concluded that in our galaxy alone there may exist as many as *forty billion* planets that could support life.

Applying some clever mathematics to their observations of these planets, the *Kepler* team learned something surprising: They discovered that planets actually deform the orbits of the very stars around which they revolve. And the denser the planet, the more it affects the orbit of the parent star.

In 1543, Nicolaus Copernicus challenged the prevailing notion that the earth was the center of the universe. In his publication *De Revolutionibus*, he presented his observations concluding that the earth actually rotated around the sun. His rejection of geocentrism was ultimately denounced by religious leaders who held to the biblical proclamation of the primacy of the earth. What followed thereafter must surely have been a debate of great intensity, with both sides fervently digging in their heels.

We now know that these seemingly irreconcilable theories are actually both right and wrong. And this paradox is elegantly resolved by the *Kepler* observations of distant planets. Like the newly discovered planets, our earth distorts the orbit of a star, our sun. Thus the delineation of master and subordinate becomes blurred. In the mutually distorting dance of sun and earth, each participant influences the other.

In the pages that follow, you will be exploring the many dances that define our species. Through metaphor and anecdote, science and educated speculation, you will gain a deep under-standing of the profound influence that our interactions with our environment have upon charting our destiny as well as our momentary well-being. And you will discover how, like our small planet's tug on the sun, each of us in turn influences all that sur-rounds us.

We humans are a polarized lot. Whether we're debating the center of celestial movement or the importance of genes versus environmental influence in human development, there is often little common ground. But now we are learning that, like plan-ets and stars, genes and environment influence each other. It has become clear that our lifestyle choices—including food, sleep, exercise, relationships, and even acts of compassion—feed back a constant flow of information to our DNA and actually modify the expression of what had been considered an immutable code. As the science of epigenetics reconciles seemingly disparate theories about our health destiny, we are learning to embrace the notion of the dance and to accept that we must design our lives accordingly.

Go Wild shows us how we can do just that, by tapping into nature's design for us. Our genetic array evolved and refined itself over millions of years to manifest health almost perfectly in response to a fairly predictable set of cues from the environment. But we've turned the tables on our life code by providing confusing social, nutritional, and chemically toxic signals. *Go Wild* reveals the depth of our current evolutionary discordance, awakening us to how our lifestyle choices foster maladaptive gene expression and thus pave the way for disease.

The mission accomplished by this wonderfully empowering book is nothing short of revolutionary. Ratey and Manning provide us with the tools we need to reestablish evolutionary concordance and eliminate the conflict that we have unknowingly created between the boundless potential imparted to each of us and the maladaptive influences that now hinder its manifestation.

—David Perlmutter, MD

GO
WILD

Introduction

Go Wild. This title at first might suggest scenes such as college kids run amok on spring break, so it's fair to ask up front: What do we mean by this? If not college kids, then maybe survivalists foraging on an island? Loinclothed hunters pitching spears at antelope or fleeing lions? We mean nothing nearly so lurid, but you're getting warmer. "Wild" is one of those overworked words with layers of loaded meanings, but we intend to strip it to its core in order to make it useful — useful even to your own personal well-being.

Our meaning is easy enough to grasp. Think of wild versus tame, wolf versus dog, bison versus cow. We have the same sort of distinction in mind now when we ask you to expand this with the somewhat revolutionary notion of applying the idea to humans. Wild humans. It's not as odd as it sounds. In fact, through deep history, through tens of thousands of years, everyone was a wild human. The very same forces that tamed wolves and made them dogs tamed humans. Call these forces civilization, and yes, obvious and abundant benefits came with the deal. We're not here to dispute those blessings. Our bedrock point has more to do with genes, evolution, and time. Human evolution occurred under wild conditions, and this made us who we are. The modern human still operates on those same genes, almost wholly unchanged. We are designed to be wild, and by living tamely we make ourselves sick and unhappy.

We are going to tell you a number of fascinating details about that design: that you are born to move with grace, born to embrace novelty and variety, born to crave wide-open spaces, and, above all, born to love. But one of the more profound facts that will emerge is that you are born to heal. Your body fixes itself. A big part of this is an idea called homeostasis, which is a wonderfully intricate array of functions that repair the wear and tear and stress of living. This ability lies at the very heart of what we mean by "going wild."

We're going to make our case by first showing you the real, sweeping, catastrophic consequences of taming. The world's leading causes of death and suffering—killers like heart disease, obesity, depression, and even cancer—are the price we pay for ignoring our genetic code, our design. But fixing this, especially fixing this on the individual level, in your life, is not as overwhelming as it sounds. That's where homeostasis comes in. The task at hand is to get out of the way and let your body's wonderfully evolved abilities for self-repair do their job. The steps are simple and doable, even in our modern world. This is not speculation. Lots of people have taken these steps, including the authors. We'll tell you about them in detail, but we also have something more planned for you. If you trace these ideas along with us through this book, we think you will come away with a new appreciation for the human condition.

One of the realizations we hope to deliver is how everything—

how you eat, move, sleep, think, and live—is connected. All of it is relevant to your well-being. This seems a simple enough idea, but it flies straight in the face of the fundamentals of Western thought, of science, and especially of modern Western medicine. The tame idea is to break down a problem into components, find out which component is malfunctioning, and fix that problem—an idea that works well enough with machines, but we are not machines. We are wild animals. The wild idea is to embrace complexity.

The fact is, your depression is not solely a condition of mind and is not isolated in the brain. It may be directly and firmly a fault of your exercise routine or choice of vegetables and protein. Your obesity may be caused by your diet or it may be linked to bacteria or lack of sleep—or, even more curiously, your maternal grandmother's low birth weight. Your failure at your job may be cured by long walks in the mountains with your dog.

Even the child's song knows that the leg bone is connected to the thigh bone; we mean to press this idea a lot further to provide some appreciation of the enormous complexity and interconnectedness of the various elements of human life.

The chapters that follow will begin to assemble the case by breaking down our various topics into subcategories, and some are the usual suspects. We will begin with the basics, by examining diet and then exercise, but that's not to say we will deliver up the usual advice. Rather, we are going to use some emerging realizations in both of these areas to establish a habit of mind, a method of thinking about the human condition. We'll build on that case by looking at a broader set of behaviors: sleep, mindfulness, tribalism, relationships, and contact with nature. As the case builds, you will notice a couple of themes. First, it will quickly become apparent that the boundaries of our categories are porous indeed. We will begin talking about nutrition, and suddenly there is a firm, physical link through an identifiable pathway to, say, brain function or the immune system. This is as it should be, because this is the reality.

But more important, you will also notice that each of these categories is a pathway, and each path leads eventually to the brain and the mind. Of course it does: the mind is the seat of well-being. Which leads us to a set of fundamentally contradictory ideas that will channel what follows. Each of these contradictory ideas is correct in its own way, and each has much to teach us.

The first of these emerges in a whole slew of statements through the years, but it's perhaps best stated in a sentence attributed to Native Americans: "Every animal knows way more than you do." The contradictory statement to this one has a long and robust tradition in Western thought, explicitly articulated even at the very root of the Judeo-Christian tradition: you, as a human, are the crown of creation, better, "more evolved," and therefore somehow separate from and superior to all other animals.

Maybe it's best to hear the first case from a field biologist, because these are often the people who, like traditional Native Americans, truly understand the idea. The act of close observation of a given species of wild animal does nothing so much as instill a deep appreciation for the inherent abilities that attune animals to the environment. The biologist was expressing this very idea to an observer one time when the observer challenged him. "Okay, if owls are so smart, why don't they build houses, cars, and computers?" The biologist's instant response was "They're so smart that they don't have to."

The same idea emerges in a more common event. You don't have to be a biologist to make a close study of an animal, and many of us do. We study our dogs. And many of us have had the experience of watching the familiar family pet deliver a litter of pups. Being proper dog surrogate parents, we research the coming event as thoroughly as possible. We make trips to the vet, we prepare for the various procedures we will need to follow to ensure each pup's first breath — there's a series of defined and specific steps to effect a clean entry into the world: clear obstructions and mucus and then stimulate, stroking gently to encourage those first few magical breaths. We think we have to, because our dog, smart as she may be, has never mothered pups before and has no access to how-to books or the instructions we printed from the Internet. And then the pups come and the supposedly ignorant first-time mother flawlessly executes each complicated step precisely as the instructions specified, and then she looks at us as if to say, "What are you here for?" The dog doesn't need to read the manual, because every animal knows way more than you do.

This is an especially important example, because it involves hormones, in this case oxytocin. Dogs have them. So do all animals, including humans, and oxytocin will figure in much of this book — even, in fact, in some surprising areas like business transactions, exercise, and violence.

But we are not restricted in thinking about instinctive knowledge of well-being in other animals, a statement that lies at the very heart of our argument. Somehow, we have gotten to the point of believing that we must ensure our personal well-being by a series of complicated gyrations and contortions, whole shelves of self-help books, multiple gym memberships, moon-launch-capable gear and telemetry, daily attention to the health section of the newspaper, support groups, and a constant count of calories. Yet imagine for a second a group of Masai men—the storied herders of Kenya—making their way across the Serengeti, an effortless trot of lithe, formed bodies, perfect conditioning, and a beauty and economy of motion that would be the envy of every dedicated gym rat. When do the Masai count calories or read the manuals? Where are their personal trainers? Or, for that matter, how do we explain the apparent well-being of the hunter-gatherer groups so assiduously studied for centuries by anthropologists and universally reported to be fit, thin, and happy? Hunter-gatherers are wild humans. Like every wild animal, they know way more than we do, which flies straight in the face of the crown of creation argument, and we do indeed mean to, at least at first, challenge that notion. Much of the damage that we inflict on ourselves, on others, and certainly on the natural world stems from extreme adherence to the notion of human exceptionalism.

Nonetheless.

The jury is still out on the question of whether the human brain is the pinnacle, the best thing evolution has ever done. The experiment has been in progress for only a couple of million years, and we have yet to see all the downsides, although a few are coming clearly into view. However, it is a simple matter of fact (and wonder) that the human brain is the most complicated and profound organ ever. In the early days of thinking about human evolution, or even today, much of what we consider exceptional about our brain is our cognitive abilities: using tools, planning, being clever—that sort of thing. These abilities are marvelous and unique. We don't mean to understate them here, but it may help to begin thinking about some other abilities as well. For instance, the purpose of all brains—not just ours, but in all sentient beings—is to allow movement, locomotion, coordination, and manipulation. We're exceptionally good at these skills as well.

Yet our cleverness, recall, learning, and grasp of fact are not all that complex as brain functions go. It turns out—and we know this because of sophisticated tools that measure and assess brain activity—that some activities we take for granted (empathy, language, and everyday social skills) are exceedingly complex; they light up the whole brain, a buzzing glow of unimaginably dense neural networks. This is what we do and what no other species can do. We'll unpack this idea slowly as we go, but know up front that what makes us human is our unprecedented ability to get along with one another. This is our crowning achievement.

And this is what interests us, but also offers a model or framework for the case we will build in the following chapters. We are going to talk about components of human activity, like diet, sleep, and exercise. But, as we have said, there are important connections among these components. More to the point, each of these activities supports the brain. Each of them in meaningful, measurable, tangible, nameable ways supports the brain and the brain's ability to light up that hypercharged network of neural pathways. These are the neural pathways that sponsor and record your well-being and ultimately your ability to connect to other humans. Light up the whole system, and you will feel better.

This book builds its case in succeeding chapters along just this path of logic. We'll begin by laying out a baseline, a summary of what we know about initial conditions and the details of human evolution. What exactly is the human condition and what is human nature? And we'll make the overarching case, by updating a more-than-century-old inquiry into "diseases of civilization," that violation of those initial conditions has made us ill. Most of what ails us today are precisely these afflictions: diseases of civilization. Then in successive chapters we'll look at the subsets of human activity: diet and exercise, sleep, tribalism, contact with nature, relationships, and mindfulness. We'll then summarize with a chapter of practical advice on the personal level.

"Wild." This is the word we need now. Before civilization, everything was wild, including humans. The polite term of anthropology is "hunter-gatherer," but calling our ancestors "wild" explains so much more. Before there was farming and cities, we were wild humans. Ever since, more and more of us have been tamed, and this is what is making us ill. All that unfolds in the following chapters will be the case for honoring the design of our bodies that evolution gave us, but the easier way to say it is this: Go wild.

Worldwide, there is a growing and necessary trend toward restoring wild systems via ecological restoration. The Europeans call this process "re-wilding." We are arguing that the human body is every bit as complex and biodiverse, it turns out, as any wild ecosystem, and like an ecosystem, it works best when restored to wild conditions. So think of this book as instructions for re-wilding your life, and maybe even an introduction to ideas that may change the way you think about life.

In the beginning, though, it may help you to imagine three scenes. You'll want to recall them every now and again throughout this book to see how different they appear. Like old-style chemical photo developing, the narrative that follows should reveal more detail in these images as our story unfolds. At first, the images will seem fuzzy and disconnected; if we do our work correctly in the pages to come, they will begin to reveal much about the human condition.

Here's one:

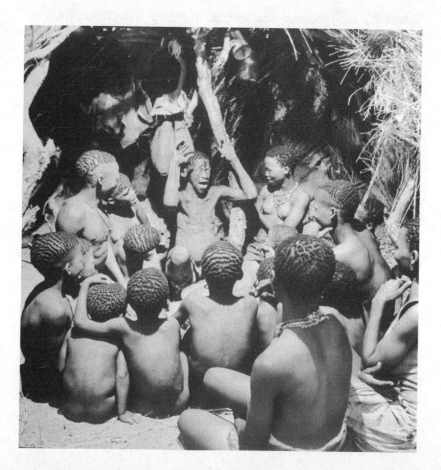

This is a photograph that we encountered years ago but that kept popping into mind as we thought about this project. There's probably a good reason it persisted, and it must begin with the fact that this is a classic photo of a band of hunter-gatherers recorded in 1947, before encroachment by civilization had compromised their way of life—and civilization did indeed make these people as sick as the rest of us in a very short time. But this is a "before" photo, and it shows a group of San people of Africa's Kalahari gathered in conversation or, probably more accurately, in storytelling, an activity that has bound us and defined our humanity for longer than we can imagine. The nakedness, of course, strikes us first, but that's a normal enough state for most of humanity for most of history. But beyond that, notice what the nakedness reveals: the lithe, fit bodies, upright and strong. Count ribs. But then check out the guy telling the story: the animation, the affect, the engagement. See what his face is doing, that he radiates a sort of magnetism that holds the circle together, engaged and involved. Who among us today communicates so well? And the circle itself? Notice that it is mostly children, that it hangs together, almost literally. There is an undeniable and readily apparent bond. There is trust.

The second image derives from a video readily available on YouTube, but anyone who has trained in developmental psychology has already seen it and heard it discussed at length, because its content explains a crucial issue of human development. But no need to go to the actual video: the scene it shows is normal enough and repeated often in every child's upbringing, at least every child lucky enough to have a reasonably normal upbringing. The scene is easy to imagine. A mother and a toddler are alone in a room full of attractions and distractions for the toddler—brightly colored toys and other objects of fascination. But it's a strange room. Toddler clings to mom but eyes attractions surreptitiously. Then courage builds, bolstered by mom's affection, and toddler leaves mom to engage an attractive object, maybe a big block. The block falls and makes a noise, and toddler immediately bolts for mom, goes through an interval of comforting, and then works up the nerve to once more go exploring, to venture off in search of the unknown.

All of this is exactly as it should be, now and from the beginning of human time. This pattern of balancing between comfort and exploration of the unknown is how we build our brains, and it is enabled by the presence of a mother's affection and support. It is the normal state of affairs, and we will need this image later, because it is not just about toddlers; it is about each of us.

The third image would at first blush seem to be about very few of us—a special case. We mean to address human well-being here as a universal, but autism is not universal. Most of us see it from afar and categorize it as one of those unlucky twists of fate that trouble a few people, maybe a genetic problem, but what has this to do with me? Yet we will build the case here that the relevance of this neurological problem goes well beyond the social costs. Autism may well be a disease of civilization, placing it right at the heart of the issues we trace here.

We were particularly struck on a visit to the Center for Discovery, in upstate New York; it's a residential facility that serves 360 people with autism, many of them too violent or disruptive to function in a normal family setting. Not all autistic people are violent or this disruptive, but the few who are wind up in places like the Center for Discovery. On the day we visited, staffers escorted us in and out of a series of classrooms, and we engaged some students without a second thought. Staffers told us that a month or so earlier this openness and access would not have been possible, that some of these people might have erupted. The staff credited the remarkable improvement in large part to an exercise regimen, and we watched people run, jump, and dance. This was their treatment: running, jumping, and dancing with one another. But just as important, this new routine built on a long-standing practice at the center of ensuring sound nutrition and connection with nature.

The scene we keep coming back to, however, was in a single tiny classroom, where four adolescent boys were seated in a row facing a simple bell and wood block that they each played in turn. A slight, dark woman with a cherubic face and a pageboy haircut sat at a small electric piano and tickled out a simple refrain, over and over again, as repetitive and simple as it had to be to engage the boys to ring the bell or strike the block, each in strict simple time to the beat laid down by the piano player. The words of the refrain echoed the activity: "Ring the bell, ring the bell, ring the bell," on and on and on. Rhythm and music, melody, meter, keeping time. This is the rhythm that calls forth a brain retreated from social engagement—the hallmark of autism.

But then we noticed the piano player, that she must perform this repetitious exercise for hours on end each day, because that is what is required of her. We noticed, too, that she was not treating this like repetition, that she was putting something of herself into each phrase, throwing in little embellishments and improvisations, that she sang from her center and, like all good singers, from the core of her emotional self. She was summoning a ray of hope to make music—not just sound, not even just melody and rhythm, but music—and doing it again and again and again in a situation that most of us would find hopeless. She was every bit as engaged and invested with the circle around her as the !Kung San storyteller. She was living the moment. She was mindful.

Appropriate, then, that this image came to us in this place, the Center for Discovery, because this was the site of one of two major turning points in each of our own stories. We have long said that there is no reason to write a book unless the process of doing so changes the author's life. Forever. Fair enough, because we hope that this book will change your life. Eventually, we will report how this happened for each of us in detail. But up front, we can say that Richard Manning lost fifty pounds and became an ultramarathon trail runner. John Ratey lost some weight, too, and changed the way he eats every day—but the big change was a major expansion in what he thinks about. He is well-known for writing about exercise and the brain, but the compelling story that is emerging at the Center for Discovery has made him far more attentive to issues like sleep, food, nature, mindfulness, and—more important—how they work together to create well-being. But it's not just the Center for Discovery that has changed John's thinking. One chance meeting, and a remarkable, spontaneous, wrenching personal account, changed his life. We'll get to that, too.

1
Human 1.0
Why Evolution's Design Endures

Evolution has hard-wired health to happiness, which means happiness is not as hard to assess as we make it out to be — not if you approach it from the wild side. Ultimately, we don't need someone else (or a book, for that matter) to define our happiness. Our brains do that. Every single aspect of the way we are wired and evolved makes it our brain's job to tell us if we are okay. Our survival depends on it being so.

Think of what our lives would be like if this were not true, if the body operated on perverse feedback loops that would tell us we are okay when we are, in biological terms, doing badly: we are hungry, cold, exhausted, and broken, and the brain says we are fine. Imagine such a feedback system, and then imagine the prospects of survival for an animal that has it. Imagine it being encoded and passed on in genes. But no need to imagine. This is precisely the perverse system that prevails in a drug addict, a hijacked system that says he is doing well when everybody can see he is not. Survival prospects? We know this answer without further study.

What we need most to understand from this is that our happiness is greatly dependent on our biological well-being, and the conditions of that well-being have been laid down by the imperatives of survival, by evolution. All of this means we need to pay attention to the conditions of human evolution to ensure our happiness. But the problem is, we don't. The popular understanding of human evolution is more or less wrong. But more important, the way we live is a clear and long-standing set of violations of the rules of human well-being, and it's making us sick.

First, summon that image that invariably pops into mind when we begin to think about human evolution: the series of cartoon panels in progression—first ape, then caveman, then us, and then a punch line. These ubiquitous cartoons make great jokes, but the idea behind them is wrong in an important way. So is the concept of a "missing link." The cartoon supports the idea that evolution gradually produced modifications and changes in human design in one neat, clear progression from our ape ancestors to who we are today, that the change was progressive, and that the process continues. All of this is wrong.

Since the time of Darwin, there has been a running debate among evolutionists, with Darwin himself taking the view that evolution was and is built on gradual transition, shade to new shade, almost imperceptibly between generations. The opposing and minority view through most of this debate has been that evolution makes sudden radical shifts, a view the controversial evolutionary biologists Stephen Jay Gould and Niles Eldredge labeled "punctuated equilibrium." The consensus now in human evolution is with the latter point—punctuated equilibrium—and we agree.

In fact, the consensus view says the package we call human, *Homo sapiens*, emerged as a whole in Africa on the order of about fifty thousand years ago. Not much has happened since. This is Human 1.0 and there have been no significant upgrades.

The consensus view was laid out by Gould himself: "There's been no biological change in humans in 40,000 or 50,000 years. Everything we call culture and civilization we've built with the same body and brain."

Yet embedded in this same cartoon and in popular understanding is a second, wrong idea, the idea of a series of links and missing links. In fact, there was not a neat line of human ancestors, each shading to the next to become more and more human-like every step of the way. The human family tree is not a towering pine with a dominant central trunk. It is more of a bush than a tree, with a series of side branches and dead ends. The most obvious example of this is the case of the Neanderthal, long known from the fossil record in Europe, Asia, and North Africa. Neanderthals are the knuckle draggers in the middle panels of the cartoon; they're also a term of insult that we use for fellow humans we consider unrefined or "unevolved," to cite one of the more egregious readings of the fundamentals of evolution. The assumption in this is clear. Neanderthals were simply a step along the way to the pinnacle, to us.

But human evolution is not a linear progression. Rather, there evolved and existed for literally millions of years—much longer than we have existed—a handful of species of viable, big-brained, upright, tool-wielding, hunting, social primates, each successful in its own niche and place. Yet modern *Homo sapiens* appear on the scene only fifty thousand or so years ago, after 90 percent of hominid evolutionary time has already passed, and suddenly we become a breakout species. Suddenly, all of those other perfectly viable hominid species are extinct, every single one. We are the only remaining species in the genus *Homo*.

Interestingly enough, there was a corresponding decrease not just in species but in genetic diversity among *Homo sapiens*. All species of *Homo*, not just *Homo sapiens*, trace their lineage to Africa. There is no serious debate or disagreement about this. And there remains in Africa some genetic diversity among *Homo sapiens*, just as one might expect in a center of origin. But beyond Africa, there is very little genetic variation in humans. There's a good explanation for this. Separation of populations is the sponsor of diversity and speciation. That is, branches occur in an evolutionary tree when some sort of usual natural event— sea level rise makes an island; glaciers divide a home range— isolates subpopulations and they begin to diverge genetically. But for at least fifty thousand years, all humans have been connected to one another through travel, trade networks, and migration. The result is a genetically homogeneous population. As a practical matter, this means when we speak of human nature, we speak of all humans, both through the time span of fifty thousand years and across the planet. Our long-standing networks of connection mean there is no pressure to drift toward a new species, no pressure to evolve.

Nonetheless, there is some variation and even innovation. Much is made of these differences among populations for deep-seated reasons having nothing to do with genetics. Take, for instance, the relatively recent experiment in light skin and blond hair. Through most of human history, maybe 80 percent of it, humans were universally dark-skinned. The experiment in light skin began in Europe only about twenty thousand years ago, an adaptation to inhabiting places with little sun. Think of how much we humans make of this tiny and insignificant blip in the total genetic makeup of our species, how much of recent human history hinges on who has it and who doesn't, "it" being a subtle little tweak not even readable in the collective genome.

Other recent experiments include such genetic variations as lactose tolerance and resistance to malaria as evidenced in a tropical disposition toward sickle-cell anemia. In this sense, we humans are evolving, but over the course of fifty thousand years, the changes have been so slight as to border on inconsequential. At least by genetic predisposition, we are no taller, no faster or slower, no smarter than were the first *Homo sapiens*. We are to the core the same guys who somehow outcompeted, outsurvived a handful of very similar upright apes to do something no other species has done before or since: inhabit every square inch of land on our planet.

But no matter how it happened, it is clear that something unprecedented took place about fifty thousand years ago. This creature called "human" appeared all of a sudden and almost as suddenly was a breakout species. The evolutionary changes that powered this breakout are the core strengths of our species and the very characteristics that we ought to pay attention to. What are these traits?

BORN TO RUN?

Start with bipedalism and running. Our habit of walking on two legs is instructive in terms of what we might gain by reexamining the issue with a fresh set of eyes.

There's a beat-up pair of Inov-8 running shoes parked under David Carrier's desk in his office at the University of Utah, and the trained eye can spot these as every bit as telling as the shape of a thigh bone. This brand is British and happens to be favored by a subset of the tribe of minimalist runners who negotiate rough mountain trails. Carrier, a trim, genial middle-aged guy with oval metal-rimmed glasses, a brush of a mustache, and a frizz of curly hair, confirms for a visitor that he is indeed a mountain runner, but this is not his claim to fame, at least in the running world, and his claim to fame in the scientific world is different still. Runners know him as the guy who tried and failed to run an antelope to death in Wyoming but then eventually figured out how to get the job done with instruction from African bushmen. Turns out it wasn't about running; it was about empathy.

Carrier's work and that of his colleagues—his mentor Dennis Bramble, also of the University of Utah, and Daniel Lieberman of Harvard—is significant beyond dead antelope to those of us who run and those of us who should run. Their findings figure front and center in a way-too-common experience: a runner consults a doctor to complain of some injury and then hears the doctor intone the sober advice, "You know, the human body is just not made for running." Thanks to Carrier's work, the runner can confidently answer, "Nonsense." Humans are in fact the best endurance runners on the planet. The best. Might this have something to do with our dominance of the planet, that we are the lone surviving upright ape?

Much is made of the fact that apes are our closest relatives, that humans are the third species of chimpanzee, and this has produced the related and wrong assumption that humans are simply apes with somehow more refined apelike features, a tweak here, a tweak there —new shades, not new colors. Yet the evidence from endurance running makes a very different case. Humans are a radical departure from chimp design.

In their pivotal paper about this in the journal *Nature*, Bramble and Lieberman analyzed the whole issue in terms of running versus walking—a way of challenging the common assumption that humans are built to walk, not run. All apes can run, sort of, but not fast and not far, and certainly not gracefully. Humans can do all of this, and this simple fact can be clearly read in our anatomical structure, in the bones. The research detailed twenty-six adaptations of the human skeleton specific to running, not walking. Some of these are, as you might expect, in the legs and feet. For instance, running requires a springy arched foot, which humans have but no other apes do. Likewise mandatory are our elongated Achilles tendons and long legs relative to the rest of the body. Running, as opposed to walking, requires counterrotation, which is to say that the upper body rotates counter to the lower, negotiated by a pivot of the hips. So running requires a far greater commitment from the upper body than walking does, and a whole collection of features designed to cope with the shifting mass.

All of these features we share with other running species, even though all of the others are quadrupeds like horses and dogs (and the fact that these two elegant runners are our closest domesticated companions through time ought to serve as a hint to the basis of the relationship). We share none of these characteristics with other species of apes—that is, with the species one limb away on the family tree. To adapt humans to running, evolution reused some older adaptations from unrelated species, and all of this took place suddenly about two million years ago with the emergence of our genus, hominids. This means that not only are we adapted to run, but running defines us.

Science has known some of this for a long time, but it was Carrier who demonstrated why this sudden departure from the rest of the ape line was so important. His working hypothesis was something called persistence hunting. True enough, many mammals, especially mammals long recognized as important food sources for humans, are terribly fast runners. Evolution takes care of them as well. But those creatures—usually ungulates like deer and antelope—are sprinters, meaning all flash but no endurance. Carrier believed that if running was so important as to deliver a watershed in evolution, humans must have used the skill to get food, persistently running game animals until they tired and faltered, and then closing in for the kill.

He gave this a try in Wyoming, where there are plenty of antelope. He found he could indeed single out an animal from the herd and track it and chase it long distances, but just as the chosen animal was beginning to tire, it would circle back to the herd and get lost in the crowd, and Carrier would be stuck on the trail of a fresh animal ready to run. Finally, though (and by chance), Carrier learned of tribesmen in South Africa who still practiced this form of hunting. He went to Africa and learned the trick, and it did indeed involve endurance running, but it also involved a sublime knowledge of the prey species and its habits, a knowledge bordering on a supernatural ability to predict what the animal would do. The running itself was meaningless without a big brain. This connection is a track worth following, but the success of the bushmen in Africa at least allowed Carrier, Bramble, and Lieberman to close their case.

Humans are indeed *Born to Run*, to cite the title of Christopher McDougall's popular book, which summarized their work.

End of the trail? Not really. In our conversation, Carrier mentioned almost none of this, and in fact took issue with some work by Bramble and Lieberman that says the human gluteus maximus buttresses the case that we are born to run. He says that the muscle in question, the butt muscle, plays almost no role in running but does show up in a host of other activities, and it is those other activities that have his attention now. He launches into a line of thought drawn from a concept pivotal in the original research — an enigma, really: a notion called cost of transport.

It's a relatively simple concept that gets straight at the efficiency of locomotion. Imagine a graph, with one axis showing speed and the other axis graphing energy expended by the creature in motion. For most species this graph forms a U-shaped curve, and the bottom of the U is a sweet spot. At this speed, the animal in question covers the most distance with the least energy, just as a car might get its best gas mileage at, say, fifty-five miles per hour. It marks the point of maximum efficiency, the best speed in terms of units of energy expended. The very existence of the U shape says that most animals have bodies meant for a given speed, a point where energy use is minimized.

Humans match the rule, but only when walking. That is, human walkers lay out a curve with maximum energy efficiency of about 1.3 meters per second. That speed uses the least amount of energy to cover a given distance. But running, at least for humans, does not produce a similar curve with a defined sweet spot; it yields a flat one. We have no optimum speed in terms of energy spent. Meanwhile, all other running animals — horses, dogs, deer—do produce a U-shaped curve when running. So if humans are born to run, where's the sweet spot? Evolution likes nothing so much as energy efficiency. Species live and die on this issue alone, so why isn't human running tuned for maximum efficiency?

Further, the whole question offers a parallel line of inquiry, not among species but within the human body itself. That's where Carrier is headed with this, but he first notes that the flat cost-of-transport curve for human running appears only when you summarize data for a number of humans. On the other hand, looking at data for each individual does indeed produce a U-shaped curve, but the sweet spot is in a different place for each human. That's not true for other species, so right off, this suggests that there is far more variability in humans, and it has much to do with individual conditioning and experience.

But more interestingly, this whole line of reasoning can be and has been examined not just between species and among individual humans but among individual muscles within a given body. Muscle recruitment and efficiency vary according to activity, even with running. Running uphill requires one set of muscles, downhill another, on the flat or side hilling different ones still. So does running fast or running slow. But further still, so does jumping. And throwing, pushing, punching, lifting, and pressing.

Carrier says that the research on this shows no favoritism, no sweet spot according to any one activity, no real specialization, and this result is counter to what's found with any other species. For other species, one can make a categorical statement like "born to gallop," but for humans, no. Born to run? Yes indeed, but also born for doing other activities as well. Humans are the Swiss Army knives of motion.

"This is not a surprise to the vast majority of people who think about what humans do, but I think it is a surprise to the folks who are so focused on the running hypothesis. We are an animal that needs to do a variety of things with our locomotive system," Carrier says. "We do more than just walk economically and run long distances."

All of this movement dictates a couple of fundamental conditions of our existence: we need to take on enough nutrients (not just energy but *nutrients*) to power all of this motion, and we need outsize brains to control diverse types of locomotion. Thinking, creating, scheming, mating, coordinating—all those activities also require big brains, but locomotion alone is enough to seal the deal. The evolution of our unique brains was locked into the evolution of our wide range of movement. Mental and physical agility run on the same track.

FUEL

There is a paradox at the center of human nutrition. All the other parts of our body seem very good at what they do, are standouts in the animal kingdom, but we are truly lousy at digestion, which is limited and puny. Literally so, because we have to be lousy at it. First off, digestion is an energetically demanding process, so why burn the calories just to take on calories if there is a better solution? But second, if we are going to be able to move around rapidly upright, we need small guts, and small guts mean short intestines, less real estate for digestion. This bit of elemental engineering is a consequence of a number of design features, but the counterrotation we talked about with running is a good case in point. Unlike all the other apes, which are quadrupeds, we have a significant vertical gap between the bottom of our ribs and the top of our pelvis, the territory of the abdominal muscles. These muscles effect the leverage necessary to keep us reliably upright and control the twist of running, so we need a light, tight abdomen, or tight abs, which restricts room for intestines.

This anatomical adjustment explains much in human makeup and behavior, but start with a simple and profound fact: our short guts mean we can't eat grass, and this is no small thing, especially if you consider that two million years of evolutionary history occurred in savannas and grasslands. Grasslands are enormously productive in biological terms; that is, they efficiently convert solar energy into carbohydrates. But that energy is wrapped in the building block of all grasses, cellulose, and humans cannot digest it, not at all.

Our primary method for overcoming our inability to digest is to outsource the job. Our prey animals, the ungulates—grazers and browsers, largely—happen to be very good at digesting cellulose. These quadrupeds can handle such tasks as chewing cuds, patiently feeding and refeeding wads and tangles of grass into a labyrinth of intestines contained in a monumental bulge of a gut.

There is no ambiguity in the fossil record, in paleoanthropology or anthropology, in everything we know about the human condition, past and present. Humans are hunters and meat eaters. There is no such thing as a vegetarian society in all the record. Eating meat is a fundamental and defining fact of the human condition, at the gut level and bred in the bones.

Discussion about this has generally been cast in terms of

protein. Essential amino acids — proteins — are necessary building blocks for that highly adapted body. The only complete source of those amino acids is meat. True as that may be, it misses some essential points, as have anthropologists and nutritionists in trying to do the calculations that explain our continued existence. When we think of meat today, we think of, well, meat, defined as muscle tissue. We disregard the rest, all those other tissues of the animal body. It's not a new mistake.

In the nineteenth century, when Europeans were exploring North America, a few explorers and fur trappers made contact with the nomadic Indians of the northern plains, a people who, like many hunter-gatherers, lived almost exclusively off animals. The Europeans of necessity adopted that diet and soon found themselves quite ill, even to the point of sprouting open, running sores on their faces. They were like we are today and ate only muscle meat. But then the Indians showed them the choice parts, the bits of liver and spleen, bone marrow and brain and the fat, especially the fat. The Europeans ate as they were told and got better because the organ tissue contained some essential micronutrients lacking in the muscle meat.

The basic energetics of an animal diet involve not just protein but also and especially fat and micronutrients and minerals, a matter of bioaccumulation. Grazers store excess energy as fat, in and of itself a dense, rich source of calories to fuel our demanding bodies; but in doing so, they bioaccumulate a rich storehouse of elements like magnesium, iron, and iodine that the deep roots of grass pull from mineral soil. This is also an important factor. Certainly we could (and do) get many of these by eating plants directly, but they are far more concentrated in meat. To get everything we need from plants, we would have to eat far more than we literally have the stomach for. Further, these minerals and micronutrients tend to be unevenly distributed on the face of the planet, as any miner for magnesium, iron, or iodine will tell you. But the big grazers tend to be migratory and range over vast areas, thereby averaging out conditions and balancing geology's uneven hand. Over time, grazing animals accumulate a full range of nutrients as no stationary plant can, and we take advantage of that life history as stored and accumulated in an animal's body.

Yet our need for variety and diversity in diet also shows up in our omnivorous habit. Humans have for all human time eaten a wide array of plants and wandered far and wide to gather them, and this, too, is more than a simple matter of energetics. Diversity ensures the range of micronutrients to support the complexity of the human body, the importance of which will emerge in detail as we develop this story. All of this gets greatly aided by our cultural adaption involving the use of fire, which allows cooking and so further aids in concentration and digestion. Add to this our microbiomes, which are another way of outsourcing to compensate for our poor digestive abilities. Our guts are loaded with thousands of species of bacteria that break down food and add value—a lot more than we think.

By and large, though, these patterns—nomadism, bipedalism, and omnivory—are defining for our entire genus and have accrued over the course of two million years of hominid history. Yet there is a variation in this theme that illustrates its refinement and gets to our more central question: the difference between Homo sapiens and all other hominids, now extinct. The general approach to food outlined here is true of all the species of hominids, even Neanderthals; yet recall that our basic question is why the single species of humans, modern humans, beat out people like the Neanderthals.

Neanderthals were indeed hunters—in fact, highly skilled hunters—and, if anything, they were more selective to very large prey animals than *Homo sapiens* were, meaning that Neanderthals had the skills and social organization necessary to kill elephants with spears. They had big hunks of protein and fat, the very thing that gave all hominids the edge. Neanderthals had bodies that were as upright and graceful as ours. They had plenty big brains. What they did not have, compared with the *Homo sapiens* of their day, was fish. More to the point, they had not learned how to tap this source of nutrition that was all around them.

Their chief competitors, *Homo sapiens*, had. Evidence of fishing first appears in Africa, but only in *Homo sapiens*. When our species showed up in Europe and Asia about forty thousand years ago, fishing of marine and freshwater sources was widespread and important on both continents.

This is not to argue that fish gave *Homo sapiens* the edge that wiped out Neanderthals, Denisovans, and *Homo floresiensis*, the other hominid species already in Asia and Europe then—although it's possible. But it does signal something important to modern nutrition, especially in the case of salmon. Remember: we can prove that those ancient *Homo sapiens* ate fish because of chemical signatures, which is to say that some elements not present in terrestrial species were present in fish, and those elements accumulate in human bones, the fossil record. Further, anyone who has ever witnessed a salmon migration, even in today's relatively impoverished conditions, understands that collecting this protein took almost no effort, as it was an almost unimaginable abundance. Forget persistence hunting: salmon eaters need only sit at streamside and rake it in, literally tons of high-quality protein. But each of those salmon, one of the world's most peripatetic species, has ranged thousands on thousands of miles across diverse marine and aquatic environments during its short life cycle. That is, each fish has sampled and bioaccumulated a diverse collection of micronutrients lacking in a terrestrial diet. Remember the value of diversity realized by nomads hunting across diverse environments. Nomads eating a nomadic marine species takes that idea up a notch: nomadism squared.

EMPATHY

The message here is diversity, and we will hear it again. But this is a small element of the larger success of humans. The details remain somewhat in dispute, but from such evidence paleoanthropologists have through the years assembled a list of traits they believe defined us as humans. In a recent book, the British scholar of humanity's roots Chris Stringer offered one such list, as good as any:

> Complex tools, the styles of which may change rapidly through time and space; formal artifacts shaped from bone, ivory, antler, shell, and similar materials; art, including abstract and figurative symbols; structures such as tents or huts for living or working that are organized for different activities (such as toolmaking, food preparation, sleeping, and for hearths); long-distance transport

of valued materials such as stone, shells, beads, amber; ceremonies or rituals, which may include art, structures, or complex treatment of the dead; increased cultural "buffering" to adapt to more extreme environments such as deserts or cold steppes; greater complexity of food-gathering and food-processing procedures, such as the use of nets, traps, fishing gear, and complex cooking; and higher population densities approaching those of modern hunter-gatherers.

It is a long list that accounts for much, but its elements, the traits, are derivative. They certainly derive from how we move, our athleticism, and what we eat and how we get it. But there are activities in here that do not derive from simple biological energetics, how we translate energy into life. Symbols (and remember: words are symbols, so this includes language)? Art? Music? Ritual? Clearly this list is telling us that something important and unprecedented has happened in our brains, something well beyond bipedalism, tight guts, voracious appetites, salmon, and the big brains that were characteristic of the hominid line for the preceding two million years.

The biologically unprecedented structures in the brain that enable these abilities don't leave much of an impression in the fossil record, so there is no hard evidence of when they appeared. We have come to know them only recently through neuroscience, an exploding field that continues almost daily with discoveries that illuminate the complexity of the brain. Yet a couple of structures, a class of cells or parts of the brain we've known about for some time, give us some hint as to why human abilities exploded on the scene fifty thousand years ago. For instance, since the 1920s, we've known about spindle neurons—a uniquely shaped set of cells that first showed up in ape brains, and to a lesser extent in dolphins, whales, and elephants, all animals known for having unique abilities. Humans have many more of them in very specific areas of the brain, and they are involved in complex reactions like trust, empathy, and guilt, but also in practical matters like planning. (You might ask why empathy and planning run together. Good question. Answer coming.)

Add to that a related and even more wondrous set of cells that neuroscientists call "mirror neurons," first discovered in the 1980s and '90s by a group of scientists in Italy. These get more to the point of empathy. The term "mirror" is apt. If we monitor a monkey's brain while the monkey is eating a peanut, the readout shows a set of firing neurons associated with activities like using a hand to pick up the peanut, chewing, and registering the satisfaction delivered by the food. But if a monkey watches another monkey eat a peanut, that same set of neurons—the mirror neurons—fire in his brain, as if he himself were the one eating the peanut. This is a major part of the circuitry of empathy, which is defined as a notch up from sympathy. More than simply realizing the feelings of another, we also literally feel them ourselves.

It would be hard to overstate the importance of this in social cohesion, but a bit of reflection shows how far this extends. It gives us some sense of another person's story, ascribing consciousness to other beings. It allows us to understand that they do not see the world as we see it, the importance of which is best understood by observing people who do not have this ability. For instance, people who have autism are notoriously altered in this very circuitry and these abilities, which is why they don't lie.

They don't see the point of lying, because they think everyone else knows exactly what they know.

This consciousness of another's point of view is exactly what enables the more elegant and refined form of lying so valuable to all humans: storytelling. It allows abstraction and conceptualization, which in turn allows language. It allows a concept of the future, which in turn opens the door to planning and scheming and is why planning is related to empathy. But it also gives us a sense that others see us, and hence body adornment shows up in the archaeological record. So does art, which is an extension of adornment but also a mode of storytelling, a symbolic representation of the world external to us.

All of this, on the other hand, comes at a great cost. As we have said, the brain is a costly organ in terms of the energy required to keep it humming along. Any additions simply increase that load, but these are more than simple additions, more than a few more cells tucked away in a discrete corner. The activities associated with spindle and mirror neurons are characterized not by the firing of a few cells but by the assembly of networks of cells all firing in concert, a glow of energy humming around the entire brain. These, unlike many of our more mundane tasks, are whole-brain activities, heavy calculation loads. This load translates into a requirement for even more calories to support it.

Yet there are more than these immediate costs involved, hinted at by one of the more intriguing and sobering bits of evidence in all the vast collection of bones: the case of a single individual, D3444. We know him only by his skull, but that's enough to tell us he was a Dmanisi man, which places his life in what is now the nation of Georgia about 1.8 million years ago. He is not even *Homo sapiens;* Dmanisi people were like Neanderthals, a separate species of hominids that left Africa long before *Homo sapiens* and eventually settled the grasslands east of what is now Europe. D3444 is a special case simply because his skull has no teeth, but, in fact, he had no teeth long before he died. Anthropologists believe this is evidence of infirmities that would have made him dependent on others for his survival. He needed help, and he got it, because hominids take care of those who can't take care of themselves and have done so since before they were humans. This generosity has real biological costs in terms of energy spent. All of this means that empathy must confer benefits greater than those costs, or it would not still be with us. This is axiomatic in evolutionary biology.

Yet any accounting of this matter can easily miss the even larger point in play. We need not look long and far for cases of humans caring for helpless humans, and this brings us to what is perhaps the most salient point of humanity, the fundamental fact of our existence largely overlooked in these discussions, because like many fundamental, important, and profound facts of life, it hides in plain sight. We take it for granted.

The biological term that we need now to move this discussion forward is "altricial," meaning simply "helpless young." Of course they are. Helpless is almost the very definition of the young of any species, from baby robins to newborn, sightless puppies. But this topic teases out probably the most significant difference between our species and all other animals now or ever. Our young are more or less helpless for a very long time, longer than any other species—fourteen, fifteen years. (Some present-day parents would insist that it's twenty-five or thirty years.) No other species is even remotely close to us in this regard. This, too, is a defining fact of the human condition.

And it is not happenstance but a predictable, derivative trait, given our big brains. Humans cannot be born with fully formed brains simply because the resulting head would not fit through the birth canal. Rather, our brains are built and formed after we are born, like a ship in a bottle, a process that takes fifteen, maybe twenty years.

Volumes of understanding and entire disciplines and sets of wisdom derive from this simple fact, but applying it to paleoanthropology offers a new lens on the human condition. In fact, some in the field now argue that this simple fact of life is the most salient characteristic of human nature, the founding fact of our life. Our young are so dependent that no parent is capable of the task of supporting and caring for that infant—not just the attention and protection, but the teaching and feeding. Hunters and gatherers must meet the energy demands of lactating mothers back in camp. Mothers simply cannot raise infants alone, and this dictates social bonding. The basic social contract has babies as its bottom line. Without this, the human species cannot go on as it is. All evolution hinges on successful reproduction of the next generation. In the case of humans, this is an enormous task. Through all human time, across all human cultures, there emerges a number associated with this task. It takes a ratio of four adults to one child to allow humans to go on. This is the real cost of our big brains.

This is why we must cooperate, and why tools like empathy and language evolved to enable that cooperation. All else of human nature is derivative of this single human condition.

Empathy and violence, tribalism and warfare, storytelling, dance, and music—all derivative. Our business as we go forward is to build the case for your well-being as it is built in humans: in mind, body, energetics, and motion, in the elements of life. But understand from the beginning that evolution—working in bone, muscle, neurons, fat, food, and fight—finally built a creature that is human. How are we different from all the rest of life? The paleoanthropologist Ian Tattersall offers a good summary. "To put this at its most elementary, humans care at least to some extent about each other's welfare; and chimpanzees—as well as probably all of our other primate relatives—do not."

Our other primate relatives did not—at least not to the extent that we do—and they are extinct.

2

What Ails Us

Not Disease but Afflictions

"Disease of civilization" is an old term that nonetheless has the power to unravel the most important questions of our time. The idea itself has been with us almost as long as the concept of evolution, yet it has taken nearly a couple of centuries for us to realize the power of linking the two ideas to explain our current disease.

But what exactly is it that ails us collectively and individually? It's not a simple or uncontroversial question, and it is one that engages a lot of scientific brainpower and serious money. There are a variety of ways to answer this, but they sort into a couple of piles, which are generally these: what kills us and what makes us sick while we are alive? The former is a problem because it runs up against the fact of our nature that we all die. Something has to kill us sooner or later, so if medical science triumphs over one cause of death, another steps in to do nature's job. We've worked around this issue with the concept of "premature death," whatever that might mean, but still, you've got to die of something. Thus we can get more traction by asking what makes us sick, what undermines our quality of life while we are alive.

It turns out that a recent and comprehensive effort to grapple with both of these aspects of the question is under way, and results will trickle out during the next few years—though the effort has already delivered some data we can use here. The Bill & Melinda Gates Foundation paid for a massive study carried out by the Seattle-based Institute for Health Metrics and Evaluation. Called "The Global Burden of Disease," it looks at causes of death but also debilitation and loss of quality of life for people suffering 291 diseases in 187 countries around the world. Further, it looks at changes in those patterns from 1990 to 2010, a snapshot of change. The first results, published in the journal *The Lancet* in late 2012, say that the world's top health problems today are, in order:

Ischemic heart disease
Lower respiratory infection
Stroke
Diarrhea
HIV
Low back pain
Malaria
Chronic obstructive pulmonary (lung) disease
Preterm birth
Road injury
Major depressive disorders
Neonatal encephalitis

More tellingly, though, these problems are related to causes, so the same study also details the top twelve risk factors for death and debilitation worldwide. Again, in order:

High blood pressure
Smoking
Alcohol
Household air pollution
Low fruit consumption
High body mass index (simply stated, obesity)
High blood sugar
Low body weight
Ambient particulate matter (air pollution)
Inactivity
High salt intake
Low nut and seed consumption

Both of these lists are telling if not surprising because of assumptions they shatter. Note the absence of cancer on the first list. Note that the list does not include, as we might expect, a litany of infectious diseases associated with poverty. The closest are malaria and neonatal encephalitis, and we can make a case that malaria is in fact a disease of civilization—just an old one. (The record shows that it only appeared with the cutting and clearing of forests associated with agriculture.) More revealing, though, is the second list: the risk factors. This is the list that undermines our concept of disease as some sort of genetic deficiency that needs to be corrected, or as simply infection by a microorganism. This list suggests that "disease" is the wrong word. What we really mean to say is "injury." Maybe it's time to abandon the time-honored phrase and begin calling diseases "afflictions of civilization."

These are not flaws or failings in the design of a person's body but, rather, self-inflicted damages brought on by the way we live. This is what ails us. Every single one of the twelve leading risk factors worldwide is a disease of civilization. But more to the business at hand: every one of these risk factors is a direct result of the foundational idea of this book. These injuries are a direct result of ignoring evolution's design of our body, a direct result of trying to force humans into conditions that the design was not meant to accommodate. And every one is easily and immediately correctable in every life. So what is the relevance of understanding nature's design of our body? Given this list, given a state-of-the-art assessment of the global burden of disease, we have a hard time imagining anything more relevant and urgent.

But you know this, or at least *can* know it. You can do your very own diagnostic of this issue without being bankrolled by Bill and Melinda Gates. Many places work well for doing this, but our personal favorite is an airport. Most any airport will do, but pick a crowded one and simply observe the stream of humanity. Obesity is what one sees first, because it is so painfully obvious; some are so obese as to require wheelchairs. Even the ambulatory are panting and sweating with the burden of a hundred-yard walk. But don't stop here. Look deeper and get some idea of everyone else's fitness, well-being, contentment (or lack), sallow sagging skin, downcast eyes. Now recall, if you're old enough to do so, the same scene in the same sort of place twenty years ago. Did it look the same? Both the numbers and your memory ought to suggest something very different. Something drastic and catastrophic is happening to our people and happening fast. We are getting worse.

Yet the irony of this fully emerges only in an airport, which is why we chose this space. What do you hear in an airport? Warnings trumpeted ad nauseam of the threat of a terrorist attack and the need for vigilance. And yet this imagined damage seems terribly meek in the face of the very real damage to our people on display before our eyes. Who did this to us? And can one imagine a greater threat to our future well-being, our future as a nation, indeed the future of our species than the condition of our people? Can you imagine an act of subversion or terrorism more powerful and more extensive than this profound injury we have inflicted on ourselves?

We can trace the concept of diseases of civilization to Stanislas Tanchou, a French physician who served with Napoleon—specifically, to some lectures he gave in the 1840s. Tanchou did not base his work on overweight people or high blood sugar; he was far more worried about cancer, as are we today. In fact, cancer was the original disease of civilization. Tanchou analyzed death registries of the day and noted that cancer was far more prevalent in cities like Paris than in rural areas, and it was on the rise throughout Europe.

By the beginning of the twentieth century, this idea had spread worldwide and had expanded to include a long list of diseases. Recall now that this was the age of imperialism, characterized by the spread of "civilization," at least as Europeans defined the term. Imperialism created a patchwork of frontiers across the globe that allowed the emerging science of the day to engage people living in the old ways, many of them hunters and gatherers. What the adventuring doctors noticed on virtually every one of those frontiers was that the so-called primitive people were in many ways healthier and more robust than Europeans. Cancer was absent in many populations around the world. For instance, a comprehensive report commissioned by America's National Museum of Natural History (part of the Smithsonian) in 1908 found cancer among Native Americans to be "extremely rare" then. One physician recorded only one case of cancer among two thousand Native Americans he examined in detail over the course of fifteen years. A population of 120,000 native people in Fiji yielded only two deaths from cancer. One physician practiced in Borneo for ten years and never saw a single case. At the same time, cancer deaths were common and well recognized (at a rate of thirty-two per thousand people) in places like New York.

Tanchou's original concept spawned a century and a half's worth of work in virtually every uncivilized corner of the globe, from Inuit, Aleut, and Apache of North America to Yanomami Indians in South America to various groups of Micronesians and Australian aborigines to !Kung San bushmen of Africa. Further, researchers began compiling a list of diseases absent in indigenous populations, no matter where they lived on the planet, including and especially cardiovascular disease, high blood pressure, type 2 diabetes, arthritis, psoriasis, dental cavities, and acne. Note that this list includes some of the very diseases that constitute our worst problems today.

Beginning as the research did in the nineteenth century, a period that made much of racial differences among people, an initial explanation for this phenomenon was, as you might expect, racist: these populations, the thinking went, were inherently resistant to these diseases by reason of what we would today call genetics. Not true. A host of studies looked at populations of these same people as they adopted Western diets and ways of living and found a coincident rise in diseases of civilization. Even the early studies showed that in those cases where indigenous people did fall prey to Western disease, it tended to occur among individuals who were living among whites. Likewise, immigration studies showed, and continue to show, that people who move from a disease-free to a disease-prone area — say from the Australian outback to Europe — quickly become as susceptible to the full range of problems as are people from that area. Diseases of civilization are not rooted in genetic differences.

A more persistent explanation emerged almost immediately in the nineteenth century and still surfaces today, a far more interesting idea tied directly to the notion that you have to die of something. In fact, some researchers signal their bias in this matter by preferring the term "diseases of longevity" to "diseases of civilization." Their argument is that the blessings of Western civilization, especially controlling communicable diseases, made people live longer and so gave them more time to develop heart disease, cancer, and type 2 diabetes. This argument stands despite a compelling counterargument: type 2 diabetes is emerging today in teenagers. So are we arguing that this is a disease of longevity caused by the fact that teenagers live longer as teenagers?

We'll be blunt, because this is vitally important to everything we will have to say, especially about nutrition: type 2 diabetes ought to be a screaming, wailing siren of a warning to our society that something is changing very fast, and we ought to do something about it. We are under attack. And while arguments and analysis may persist in complicating this problem, it is not at all complicated. Type 2 diabetes is a lifestyle disease that results from eating sugar and refined carbohydrates. It appeared among the earliest recorded diseases of civilization, coincident with sugar and flour appearing in people's diets in places as distinct as Africa and Arizona, and has been with us for more than a century. But this is not a static story.

A generation ago, doctors training in the United States would welcome the arrival of a case of type 2 diabetes, simply because it was so rare. Any walking, talking case presented an opportunity for hands-on experience. Among children, type 2 diabetes was then nonexistent. The problem began turning up more often in the general population, and then only after a lifetime of sugar eating had a chance to fully develop into the obesity that tends to run in tandem. Today, the disease is epidemic among American teenagers, especially poor American teenagers whose diet is dominated by nothing so much as sugar. To cite a news report from 2012:

> The percentage of U.S. teenagers with "pre-diabetes" or full-blown type 2 diabetes has more than doubled in recent years—though obesity and other heart risk factors have held steady, government researchers reported Monday.
>
> The good news, the researchers say, is that teen obesity rates leveled off between 1999 and 2008—hovering between 18 percent and 20 percent over the years.

The spread of diseases of civilization is a continuum that stretches into our time, an epidemic that took a couple of centuries to build. It began with imperialism but has exploded today. Calling these diseases of longevity misses a crucial point, but longevity is indeed relevant in this context, and to explore this idea, we need a more refined picture of longevity among hunter-gatherers. The contention that they all died early is nothing more than an extension of the Hobbesian idea that life before civilization was nasty, mean, brutish, and short. Indeed, the average life expectancy of many hunter-gatherers was probably lower than ours. That's not to say that some of them did not live to a ripe old age; plenty of anthropologists' accounts record old people as valued and active members of tribes. They could live long, healthy lives. The average, nonetheless, was skewed by a number of factors, especially high mortality among infants and young people. In biology among all species in the wild, high mortality of young individuals is the norm, and humans were then living in the wild.

Still, there's an important extension of the record of this issue that speaks to the overall quality of life, longevity, and well-being of our ancestors. This inquiry into diseases of civilization is not at all restricted to the past couple of centuries. The imperialism and colonization of the nineteenth century was only the culmination of a process that began with the advent of civilization—by which we mean the advent of agriculture—about ten thousand years ago. That longer period produced a much longer record, and the evidence is clear. North America provides one of the best examples.

The general notion of pre-Columbian Native Americans is that all of them were hunter-gatherers like the archetypal bison hunters of the Great Plains. Yet by the time Columbus arrived in the New World, hunter-gatherers were as rare in North America as they were in, say, Eastern Europe at the same time. By and large, Native Americans of 1492 were farmers, settled agricultural people, but there were, at the same time, pockets of hunter-gatherers across the landscape. Paleoanthropologists have examined skeletal remains of both groups in detail and found general agreement with the record worldwide and through time. The hunter-gatherers were taller, less deformed, showed no evidence of diseases of civilization like dental cavities and no deformation of their bodies; but the skeletons of the contemporaneous Native American farmers revealed all of these problems. Native Americans showed evidence of suffering diseases of civilization long before Western civilization arrived, which is why we need to define civilization as the arrival of domestication, of agriculture. We are really talking about diseases of agriculture and adoption of the sedentary way of life.

Now we have arrived at the point in this argument that, according to established ritual, requires an insertion of a disclaimer, the "yeah, but..." These discussions generally become defensive, as if anyone raising these ideas is attacking the very core of civilization and advocating a return to living in caves. It is true enough that despite the costs, civilization came with considerable benefits: our kids don't die as often now, and we need not fear infection (as much) or a full load of body parasites. The disclaimer is indeed warranted but nonetheless misses the point. The costs associated with civilization, the diseases of civilization, are to some degree reversible. By paying close attention to what lies at the root of this series of problems, we can erase some of these costs. We can learn from our ancestors to steer our way to well-being. And it turns out that while these issues in all their layers are as complex as civilization itself, the root, the one central development that gets us to maybe 80 percent of what ails us, is simple: it is glucose and glucose alone, in all its permutations. In the end, this discussion will gather threads as diverse as violence, infant attachment, tribalism, meditation, and dance, but we must begin with glucose, because that's where civilization began.

IT'S THE GLUCOSE

In many ways, it took ten thousand years of gradual change to mold us in the shape we are in today. We like to fault modern industrial agriculture and everything that goes with it — overpopulation, a hyperindustrialized food chain, and sedentary living — as underlying the epidemic sweep of diseases of civilization. But the fact is, these all began millennia ago, when humans first domesticated grain. This is a bedrock belief among anthropologists. The effects of the Industrial Revolution and the Information Age pale in comparison with the effects of the advent of agriculture, the single greatest change in two million years of hominid history. So profound were its effects on humanity that it has been said it makes every bit as much sense to argue that wheat domesticated us as the more usual and opposite statement.

Yet it's wrong to say that humanity has been living under agriculture for ten thousand years and that it all traces to wheat. Wheat was simply the Western side of the story. True enough, agriculture did begin with the domestication of wheat about ten millennia ago, but early farming was far more integrated with hunting and gathering for several thousand years and did not do much to reorganize the human endeavor until maybe six thousand years ago in the areas that are now Iraq and Turkey. Further, agriculture also began with independent domestication of separate crops in a continuous process stretching to maybe five thousand years ago, with the domestication of rice in Asia and Africa, maize in Central America, and tubers like potatoes in South America. All spawned separate civilizations, but crucially, except for the South American case of potatoes, all were based in the taming and cultivation of a wild grass (yes, rice, wheat, and corn, or maize, as most of the world knows it, are grasses), and all, including the tubers, rested on plants that stored dense, durable packages of carbohydrates: starches. This is civilization. Civilization is starch, and by extension, diseases of civilization are diseases of starch, either directly or indirectly, and most of it is indeed direct: starches are complex carbohydrates, and they quickly break down, often even in a person's mouth, into simple carbohydrates, which are sugars. Further, much of that sugar is glucose or other forms that the liver converts into glucose.

The human body is perfectly capable of metabolizing glucose, which has been with us through the ages, especially in fruits and tubers. We convert it into glycogen, and any athlete will tell you that glycogen is what moves us forward. (It turns out that this is not nearly as true as we think, but for the moment, let's let this stand.) It is not that glucose is unprecedented or even that starch is new to us; hunter-gatherers have and had both. But not in abundance, not as a sole source, not in the tidal wave of starches that agriculture would begin yielding ten thousand years ago, a wave that has built exponentially in our time.

Today, those three wild grasses — rice, wheat, and corn — are the three most dominant forms of human nutrition, and the potatoes domesticated in South America are the fourth. About 75 percent of all human nutrition derives from those four sources alone. To oversimplify just a bit, this is what ails us, and we will unpack this idea in the next chapter, where we'll look at the diseases of civilization clustered around metabolic syndrome, the most important and most devastating of these ailments. Reversing this is where we can begin reversing the worst effects of the way we live. In effect, this is the reversal of domestication, which is to say the first step in going wild. Still, this issue does not end with glucose, obesity, and type 2 diabetes.

Dense packages of storable starch allowed sedentary lives. That is, we no longer needed to range far and wide as nomadic hunter-gatherer societies had done for a couple of million years; we could spend our lives in a single location—or, as this tendency has played out in modern times, in a single chair. Domestication allowed cities. Domestication created new sources of protein but also new sources of disease, because most of our infectious diseases come from domesticated animals, especially chickens and swine. Storage of grain, though, also allowed accumulation of wealth, almost immediately accruing preferentially to a few individuals. Evidence of disparate wealth is abundantly clear in the archaeological record in the very first agricultural cities, yet it's unknown in hunter-gatherer societies, both in the archaeological record and among contemporary wild people. By allowing wealth, civilization, by extension, created poverty.

Grain allows soft food for infants, and a sedentary life allows women to begin producing children earlier and more often, which is to say that grain greatly accelerated population growth.

These are the most cited and most obvious effects of domestication. The more subtle implications are just as interesting. For instance, remember that we began by talking about cancer, which develops from a complex set of circumstances through lifetimes. The story of cancer and civilization yields to no simple telling, but a quick look at one small example is illustrative and important in its own right, especially to women: the epidemic rates of breast and ovarian cancer in our time. But how does this relate to evolution and agriculture?

Evolution is profoundly attentive to a couple of issues: food and reproduction—how we survive day to day and through generations. Nothing is more important to evolution as a trait that speaks to *both* food and reproduction.

The human body has a long list of mechanisms for assessing well-being, and nowhere are these more important than in reproduction. Science has clearly demonstrated that the body's sensory systems have highly developed ways of ensuring that babies are born during times of plenty, during times of maximum well-being. The normal time of onset of a first menstrual period for a hunter-gatherer girl is about seventeen years old, which is somewhat surprising for anyone following the corresponding number among modern girls in postindustrial societies. Menarche for this latter group is more like twelve years old.

There is plenty of speculation as to why this is true. Genetic differences? Nope. There are many studies showing, for instance, that when Bangladeshi girls move to England as children, their first periods come at the normal time for English girls, not Bangladeshi girls. Can polluting chemicals and endocrine disruptors or food additives explain this phenomenon? There may well be an effect, but there is a simpler and well-researched explanation: body weight. The fatter a population, the more likely a girl is to menstruate early. Hunter-gatherer girls were and are lean and active and so develop according to nature's long-term plan. Carbohydrates and sedentary habits in domesticated populations circumvent that plan, simply because such girls are fatter and the body's sensors rightfully detect flush times. Time to reproduce.

The real downside of this (other than rampant teenage pregnancy, and we hope that you see in our reasoning that we think the coincidence of the epidemic of obesity and teen pregnancy among impoverished girls is more than a coincidence) comes at the end of life, though. Menarche launches girls into a regular cycle of hormones. The result is that any girl who starts early and has a lifetime of menstrual regularity with few pregnancies (lean, athletic girls and women often do not menstruate regularly) has approximately twice as many periods and so twice as many bouts of hormone cycling as hunter-gatherer girls. One of those hormones, progesterone, triggers cell division, and because both breasts and ovaries take strong doses twice as often, those become sites of tumors. This is how both breast and ovarian cancer appear as diseases of civilization. Researchers have examined this and suggested an interesting intervention for both forms of cancer: an exercise program for girls. We agree.

AUTOIMMUNE

The Tsimané people are a surviving population of hunter-gatherers in Brazil's Amazon rain forest. Doctors studied twelve thousand Tsimané extensively, a total of thirty-seven thousand examinations, and found what, by now, we might expect. No cancer of breast or ovary, but no colon or testicular cancer either. Cardiovascular disease? Absent. No asthma. Zero. One more fault of carbohydrates? Not really. Not directly. Asthma opens a new and fascinating door, and through it we enter a whole new area, a second wave, if you will, of diseases of civilization, one that ought to raise our appreciation of the intricacy of evolution to something approaching awe.

Asthma is an autoimmune disease, and the Tsimané people have about one-fortieth the rate of autoimmune disease as do the people of New York City.

An autoimmune disease is, in simplest terms, an example of the body attacking itself. Something relatively benign, a foreign body but not a real threat, triggers an immune response, and this powerful system suddenly launches the body's equivalent of all-out thermonuclear war, like a trigger-happy paranoid. This is our new epidemic, what the science writer Moises Velasquez-Manoff aptly labeled "an epidemic of absence."

First, the problem is indeed epidemic. Run-of-the-mill infectious diseases like rheumatic fever, hepatitis A, tuberculosis, mumps, and measles are all in decline worldwide, declining in some cases from universal in 1950 (everyone then got mumps and measles) to nearly zero today. In that same period, autoimmune diseases like multiple sclerosis, Crohn's disease, type 1 diabetes, and asthma have at least doubled, in some cases quadrupled.

Second, the epidemic is very new, appearing only in the last generation, and it followed an even more intricate but parallel path to that of diseases of civilization. All the autoimmune diseases showed up first and most markedly in people living at the very pinnacle of civilization, in cities, and in the best areas of cities at that. Penthouse dwellers on the Upper East Side got asthma. Alabama hog farmers did not.

The "absence" part of the characterization, however, is even more interesting. The standard explanation for the prevalence of autoimmune diseases is an idea dating to the 1980s. It suggests that autoimmune diseases are a direct result of our success in eradicating not only bacteria that cause infectious diseases, but also parasites like hookworms.

Velasquez-Manoff summarized the matter: "Immune-mediated disorders arise in direct proportion to affluence and Westernization. The more that one's surroundings resemble the environment in which we evolved—rife with infections and lots of what one scientist calls 'animals, faeces and mud'—the lower the prevalence of these diseases."

This is where the argument gets evolutionary or, more to the point, coevolutionary, a term coined by the conservation biologists Paul Ehrlich and Peter Raven. The hypothesis of coevolution says simply that when species evolve in the presence of each other, in a long-term relationship, removing one can damage the other, even if they are bitter enemies, like wolves and elk or infectious bacteria and humans. It is a rule that says even well-intentioned interventions in natural systems can have profound deleterious consequences. This idea, in fact, is getting some traction among researchers, and today consideration of the human microbiome—the population of microbes that inhabits every human body—is becoming one of the hottest pursuits of medicine. It's a truly positive development.

The mechanism that produces the epidemic of absence in the case of autoimmune diseases is fairly straightforward, and also evolutionary. Toward the end of the Paleolithic era, as glaciers advanced and pushed a growing human population into a more restricted area, even before farming began, there was an increase in a few infectious diseases like malaria. Over time, evolution adjusted and favored those humans with the most reactive immune systems, and there are specific, known genes for this. The most interesting case study was in Sardinia, an island off of Italy, which was in this period and until modern times plagued by malaria. Researchers found a prevalence of genetic fitness in the population of Sardinians. Selection pressure made them highly effective at defeating malaria. The phenomenon was so finely tuned that people in coastal areas had this fitness and people who had long lived a few miles away in the highlands (where there was no malaria) did not. But Sardinia, like many countries, wiped out malaria in the twentieth century, and then those hypertuned, aggressive immune systems went looking for a new enemy, like an overmuscled bully stewing for a fight. As is often the case, the new target was the body itself. Sardinia today has epidemic levels of the autoimmune disease multiple sclerosis. This is the very pathway that shows up in all the other autoimmune diseases that plague us today in ever-increasing numbers.

We have approached this whole topic as a separate front in the advance of diseases of civilization, but there are in fact interesting connections between the first and second waves, some cross talk between food and immune response. Know that this is not simply a matter of an oddball infectious microbe that we happen to encounter. Microbes are not at all incidental to our lives, an idea that we hope will give you a new way of thinking about yourself as not just yourself. The thing is, you have more microbes, mostly bacteria, inside of you right now than there are humans on earth. Bacterial cells inside you outnumber your own cells, and the genetic code of the raw information of the microbes that you contain dwarfs your own genetic code. Yours is a thumb drive to their terabytes of hard drive.

Do you think nature would use all of that information for nothing, or that those uses have nothing to do with your health and well-being?

Consider raw energetics, for instance. Remember: we humans need all the help we can get to boost our streamlined digestive system, and clearly we use microbes for this very reason. An argument we will make later on is that the often-cited dictum of traditional nutrition that says a calorie is a calorie is just plain wrong. Some research has shown that the calorie content made available to your body is, in fact, to some degree dependent on the type of bacteria in your digestive system, a population that varies wildly from person to person. But in a marvelous display of symbiosis, what happens typically is the bacteria in your digestive system live off your food — that is, they take the energy they need, and at the same time make some energy more available to you, increasing energy content by, on average, 10 percent. There is a species of bacteria found in obese mice that, when transplanted into other mice, makes them obese. Same diet. New bacteria, and they become obese. There is some evidence that certain bacteria give us vitamins we wouldn't normally extract from food. But even "good" bacteria can go bad in interesting ways.

For instance, in one experiment, researchers fed normally lean people a diet of junk food and noted a flourishing of a species of bacteria that caused the subjects to harvest even more calories from the junk food and in turn grow more obese. But because these are bacteria, they are of interest to our immune systems, and immune systems sometimes respond to invasions with inflammation. We will have a lot to say about inflammation as this book goes on, but know that many researchers now

worry far more about inflammation than they do about cholesterol in the origins of heart disease, not to mention cancers. In
the junk food experiment, those flourishing junk food bacteria
produced a marked increase in both inflammation and insulin
resistance, which is the indicator at the dead center of diseases
of civilization.

Yet all of this merely scratches the surface of a largely unex-
plored universe. Our bodies contain thousands of species of bacteria, each with the potential to affect our well-being in direct
ways; we know almost nothing about them, and yet we, for generations, have not hesitated to introduce tidal waves of upheaval
into our internal biomes with routine doses of antibiotics.

Further, once this complex system has been so disturbed—
and there is no doubt it has been in each of us—we still have
not the foggiest clue as to how to put it back together.

A generation ago, scientists working in another field (literally a field) faced a similar problem, and it offers an informative
analogy, perhaps even an exact parallel. The issue was simple
enough that a few conservation biologists hatched plans to con-
duct what was then called restoration ecology: the idea of restoring intact ecosystems. That's the first step in connecting you to
this analogy. You are not an individual so much as you are an
ecosystem. Your health and well-being depend on the health of
that ecosystem. You confront the exact same problem of restoration ecology in your internal biome.

These biologists faced a challenge, and prairie restoration,
then and now popular in the American Midwest, was a good
example. They encountered a plowed, fertilized, sprayed farm
field and wondered how to restore the complex array of plants,
animals, and microbes that once made it succeed so magically as

prairie, with literally hundreds of species of plants working in concert.

They often would start out by simply cataloging the species of plants that they knew should be there; then they would get seeds and start planting the desired species, often discovering that target species would not grow. A prairie is a complex ecosystem and cannot be so straightforwardly engineered. What they got after planting, it turned out, was highly dependent on initial conditions and the unimaginably complex interplay of all the species in question. Often they found, for instance, that they needed fire, roaring, scorching fire, and often they found that they didn't need seeds. Once conditions were right, dormant seeds, some dormant for centuries in the soil, sprouted and flourished.

We face something like this in understanding how we restore our personal ecosystems, and, in fact, all the leading health-food stores are perfectly happy to offer you "probiotic" supplements, designed to replace this bacterium or that. There is no evidence that these work, that the species being sold is absent in you, or that this species will flourish, given existing conditions in your personal ecosystem, your microbiome. This is a more complex matter. Just as with prairie, it is not a simple matter of having the right seeds.

And yet we can't help but think that appreciating the complexity of the task at hand is itself enlightening, not just in matters of bacteria and autoimmune diseases but in everything we have to say about restoration of your body and mind. Above all, you are complex—too complex not to suffer some ill effects from all the tinkering civilization has wrought on your body. This nicely frames the task at hand.

3

Food

Follow the Carbs

These days George Armelagos can be found as often as not in a first-floor office of Emory University's Anthropology Building, although it does not look exactly like an office—more a wonderful mess. The place is strewn end to end with layers of books, papers, and generations' worth of academic accretion of near-archaeological proportions. A large, square plastic wall clock advertising Coca-Cola (we are in Atlanta, after all, corporate headquarters of the empire of sugar water)—the sort that one would expect to find hanging on the wall of a burger joint— stands on a desk. It doesn't work.

Armelagos's walker is parked to one side and the man himself has eased into a low chair behind the desk. He wears a weathered purple polo shirt two sizes too big, with no attention paid to the buttons. A pile of long black hair with strands headed in most directions rings his bald spot. He's seventy-eight and has a bit of a struggle getting around, but he carries a teaching load and commands the long view of the topic at hand. Years of thinking about what we ought to eat rests on some of the work he did in the

1970s, back when no one had really thought seriously about these matters, when no one challenged our most deeply seated prejudice about the manifest blessings of civilization. Back then, Armelagos thought civilization was a blessing, too.

Armelagos is an anthropologist but only deflected in that direction after signing on to the University of Michigan's medical school, a solid path for a Greek kid from Detroit in the 1950s. His academic pathway made him interested in bones, and he has been a bone guy ever since. Once he was in anthropology, med school gave him something of a leg up, in that there was bone work to be done. And, in fact, his colleagues were engaged in intriguing questions about mortuary practices, such as the detailed study of the angle of the head and the curl of the leg in ancient North American burial mounds. He had the notion, though, that bones might also offer some guidance on what were then viewed as less pertinent questions, such as about the health and well-being of the living.

In the late '70s, Armelagos set his sights on the Dickson Mounds, the leavings of a Native American culture that once lived along the Spoon River in Illinois. The mounds themselves were surviving evidence of a culture of about fifteen hundred years ago, in a period of transition. That is, they recorded a crucial event, the transition to agriculture—the corn and bean agriculture that was the mainstay of pre-Columbian North America, from Mexico northeast along a broad band stretching to the Atlantic coast and north into what is now Ontario. The Dickson Mounds held the bones of these people, but also nearby were remains of the hunters who had lived in the same area, the primitives who preceded the farmers. The working hypothesis of the day was that people around the world, not just in North

America, grew in numbers to the point of decimating game supplies, and so suffered famine, famine that sent them to agriculture and its greater productivity. And then they got healthy again, or so Armelagos and everyone else at the time thought. That assumption was also a testable hypothesis, given the bones at Dickson, so Armelagos set out to test it.

He began by looking at infectious diseases and expected those to be a negative effect of civilization. The more closely people live together, the more likely they are to become infected with disease, and even then, science acknowledged this as a cost of civilization.

"We expected to find an increase in infectious disease rates, but we didn't expect to find an increase in nutritional deficiencies. That was really counterintuitive," he said.

The evidence, though, was clear. The farmers were less well fed, more deformed, and shorter than the hunters who had preceded them.

To be fair, Dickson was probably an extreme case. Early farmers there probably had only corn, and later adopted the beans that provided some of the nutritional balance in this system of agriculture. Still, there has been a broad repetition of this line of inquiry ever since. Similar sites worldwide tell a story of the transition to agriculture that's consistent with the overall picture at Dickson. The record does indeed show that there were hunter-gatherers who suffered health problems from nutritional deficiencies, but these are exceptions. The overall record, the broad story, says civilization was a mixed blessing. It came with enormous costs to our health, and at the beginning, most of those costs were directly tied to a decline in nutrition. Agriculture brought malnourishment.

Armelagos started publishing his findings in the late '70s, leading to a couple of pivotal books, including *Paleopathology at the Origins of Agriculture* (coedited by Mark Nathan Cohen), long out of print but republished by popular demand in 2013. Colleagues of his at Emory University—Melvin Konner, Marjorie Shostak, and S. Boyd Eaton—cited Armelagos's work in *The Paleolithic Prescription* in 1988, which is the genesis of the current paleo diet trend, the line of thought that carries forward to today's popular diet books by authors like Loren Cordain. Along the way, the idea has become a movement of sorts, complete with schisms, disciples, true believers, and dogma. Today there are even "paleo" sections in supermarkets and a magazine dedicated to the whole business.

And to compound matters, paleo does not stand alone as the sole thread of this idea. A second strain follows the low-carbohydrate banner, beginning with the Atkins diet and extending through prescriptions like the Zone and fat flushing. The unifying idea of these two strains was to shun carbohydrates, especially the refined sort that arrived with agriculture.

Armelagos has watched all of this transpire with some bemused fascination and has commented in one paper: "A number of these studies follow rigorous scientific methods and have been highly influential in shaping what we know about variety, change, benefits, and costs of prehistoric diets. Unfortunately, these scholarly works have been used to create numerous popular publications that claim some degree of scientific validity."

He cites a reductio ad absurdum of this trend: a volume popular in some circles titled *What Would Jesus Eat?*

So what would Armelagos eat? He has a couple of ready answers to this, answers he believes properly reflect his original findings but also everything we have learned since. And his prescription is a lot simpler than you might think, boiling down to two crucial points. We cite them here because we agree. One is obvious, though it is not at all trivial: low carbs. The second is less talked about, but in Armelagos's thinking and ours, the second is even more important: variety. But understand first that these problems did not end with the demise of the people at the Dickson Mounds.

CASE STUDY

By the strangest of coincidences, our hunting and gathering for this book led us to a story of a young woman in Alpena, Michigan, who had suffered a remarkable string of health problems. And unremarkable in a way, because Mary Beth Stutzman, it turns out, had a lot in common with a lot of us—not just in her problems but in her encounter with our health-care system. So we tracked her down and let her tell her story in her own words. What follows is a transcript of a conversation recorded on May 29, 2013. It has been edited only for length. We wanted you to hear her story in her words, because of its relevance to the topic at hand, but also for the underlying themes that will recur throughout the book.

MARY BETH STUTZMAN

I am thirty-four right now, so going back to when I was about nineteen or twenty is when I first started noticing that I was having some issues. I was always a skinny kid. I never worried about weight. I could eat a whole bag of Hershey's Kisses and I did not gain an ounce. I grew up on a farm, so we would always eat good and fairly healthy.

I was getting ready to move away from home and go to school at Michigan State [University]. I started having bad stomach pain. It felt like my stomach was cramping. It lasted for weeks. It was really painful, like something inside was being twisted. I went to the doctors, and they said they were not sure what was happening. They said maybe you have an ulcer.

I started to not be able to sleep at night. I developed really bad acne. There were things that were unusual, but looking at them individually, I was a college student. I was very driven and ambitious. I was working while going to school. It is not uncommon that college kids have trouble sleeping, so I didn't think a whole lot about it.

I started having other problems with my stomach. I couldn't digest any food. I would start eating and feel bad. This was independent of the other stomach pain. All of a sudden, I would feel so bloated I couldn't take it anymore, and I would just vomit everything I had eaten the whole day fully undigested.

It was really hard to sleep at night, and some days I would just never fall asleep. I would have to go to work the next day, and it would make me feel like I had the flu for the whole day. After about five days of that, I would have to take a day off from work, go home, rest, and hope that I would fall asleep. It was getting to the point where one night Casey [her husband] and I were watching TV. A documentary came on about insomnia, and I started crying because I was so frustrated with myself [for] not being able to sleep.

I had tried all the home remedies, I had gone to a therapist, and people thought I was just a highly depressed person. I didn't think so, but that was what people were saying, so I thought, oh, I have to do something, so I tried meditation. I exercised regularly. I was running about three to four miles per day and lifting weights so I wasn't out of shape. It was really strange. So I went to the sleep clinic and I did the study. They said you don't have sleep apnea or anything like that. Your brain is hardwired to always be active.

After that, I tried maybe six different sleeping pills and an antidepressant to try to find something that would help me sleep, and nothing worked. This was over the course of another five years. I tried all these different things. I would try one for six months. It wouldn't work. I had bursitis in both of my hips. I was twenty-five when I went to the doctor about that. It is like an arthritic condition. What twenty-five-year-old gets arthritis?

So now we come up to the point where I'm pregnant. I had a whole lot of problems with pregnancy. I gained about seventy-five pounds. This was the first time in my life I gained any real substantial weight [in] more than a five-pound increment. I had postpartum depression. More problems with my stomach. I went in and had a CAT scan, and they said that parts of my intestines were becoming paralyzed. They put me on a liquid diet for three days, and then after that I could eat soft foods like mashed potatoes.

I struggled to take the weight off. I did boot camp after boot camp. I only lost two pounds. I cut back on crap in my diet. I hadn't eaten chips in forever. I didn't drink a lot of pop. I was following a very healthy diet. I had whole grains at every meal. I was eating vegetables and having meals plus snacks to keep my metabolism going. I was working out hard, at least an hour a day at least five days a week, and I was not losing a single pound.

Oh, and then the asthma. Asthma all of a sudden became a problem, and I had to carry an inhaler, and bursitis was still an issue.

No one suggested these things were connected, and no one suggested that I should look at my diet. No one ever mentioned it. I went to my family doctor, who had been seeing me since I was a kid. I went in with a list, and I had handwritten notes, both sides of pieces of paper covered with notes. I said I have been dealing with a lot of stuff, and I have been coming in individually for things, and they are not really getting any better. They are actually persisting, and I think all I am doing is learning how to cope with them.

I took in two pictures of myself. I said look at these two pictures. I know I look kind of the same [in each], but when you look at my face, right now my face looks bigger, and it looks like it's changing. I know your face changes as you get older, but mine looks longer, doesn't it? He looked at me, and he said, "Have you ever seen a therapist for your problems?" It was said with a tone that I am surprised I didn't start crying right there. But I was like, oh my God, I don't know who else to go to.

So he left the room to go and schedule an MRI with the nurse, and he didn't close the door all the way, and I heard the nurse say, "What? You want what? For heaven's sake, have you seen the list that girl has? It's two pages long. We are going to be here all night. I don't have time for this."

I was feeling like maybe I was making a big deal out of nothing. Maybe I'm too whiny. Maybe everybody feels this way, and

I'm not handling it well. It was just frustrating, and I kind of gave up a little bit for a little while.

I never felt rested. I started waking up, like, three times in the middle of the night having seizures, but with my whole body convulsing. I would wake up in the middle of them, and after a few minutes, they would go away, and I was conscious. It was very strange. I didn't go see the doctor about them because I was busy, and other stuff was happening, and I was so sleep-deprived, I was just trying to make it through every day. I had no energy to do anything, even though I was forcing myself to work out. I thought: Maybe if I could work out more. I'm not doing it enough. This is supposed to give you energy. Maybe I'm not doing it right. My husband is a personal trainer and he was helping me.

I remember sitting on the toilet one day, trying to have a bowel movement and nothing was happening, and this was after about five days. This was normal. I would go seven times in one day, and then I wouldn't go for a week. I remember I had the feeling it was growing [worse]. It was not anything that I noticed right away, but then it became really clear that something else was happening.

I made an appointment with a new doctor. I said stuff was going on, and I didn't really know why, and I talked with her about it. I said I would really like to start exhausting my possibilities. I told her, if you're willing to work with me, I want to have every test done because something is going on, and I don't know what, but I can't live like this anymore. She said, "Okay."

I started getting a migraine headache during the appointment, and within about ten minutes, I couldn't talk because the headache was so bad. It turned out it was just a normal migraine, and they sent me home with pain medication for the headache. After a day or two I recovered, and I just got back to my normal making-it-through-the-day routine.

A few days later, I have another migraine coming on. I get my daughter in the car, and I'm driving her, and it's getting worse and worse by the second. It had never come on so fast before. I'm starting to get worried. I go through the busiest intersection in town. The light is green, and I have to throw up. I couldn't stop. I didn't want to cause an accident, so I open my door and throw up on the street. I get through the light, and I have to stop and throw up again. I threw up all over my steering wheel, my seat, my lap, the floor, and the radio.

A couple of days after that, I'm not doing too bad, and we had plans to go on this cross-country ski trip. I hadn't been cross-country skiing since I was a kid, so I was excited. I was looking forward to it. We go skiing, and everyone leaves me in the dust. I was the slowest person there, despite the fact that I exercise regularly. I was behind everyone.

That night my stomach hurt like it had never hurt before. I just couldn't take it anymore. I had been getting up at night. I wasn't able to sleep, so I was getting up out of bed and trying to walk. I remembered growing up on the farm and having horses with colic. I couldn't walk without poking my fingers into my side where my colon was; it hurt so much.

Finally, about two or three in the morning, I woke Casey up, and I said, "I don't know what is going on but it never hurt this bad before. I have to go to the ER." I got there, and they put me in a room. They had me drink some stuff, gave me a CAT scan, and they took an X-ray. It comes back, and they said, "Your intestines are paralyzed in three different areas," and they showed me: here, here, and here. "Your colon is not working at all. We are not sure what is causing this, but you have stool backed up all the way to your small intestine." The doctor said, "You are one sandwich away from a ruptured bowel, which can be deadly. We need to get this out of you right now." In the X-ray, my colon was extended all the way up into my rib cage below my heart.

So that evening I had five enemas to try to clean out my system. I had never had one before. It was embarrassing. I felt completely humiliated, but at the same time, I was willing to do whatever it took to get me back home.

They put me on a liquid diet. I spent two, almost three weeks keeping myself alive with soup broth and Ensure shakes that old people drink. That was all I could handle. I couldn't eat real food. That would hurt too much. I remembered when I used to do marketing for the hospital, and I interviewed a cancer patient one time who had throat cancer and couldn't eat solid food. His wife said she had researched how many Ensure shakes he would need to drink each day in order to have enough calories and nutrients to stay alive, and that is what she did. This guy survived for a year drinking Ensure shakes. I thought to myself, no big deal. I can drink Ensure shakes and keep myself alive.

I went to a gastroenterologist and had more tests that basically said the same thing. They thought for sure that I had Crohn's disease, and the entire conversation centered on verifying that I had Crohn's disease. They did a colonoscopy of my lower intestine and bowel, and they found no evidence of Crohn's. There were no lesions. There was no scarring. Nothing. All they found was severe inflammation, which they said was not an issue.

My dad drove me to the appointment, and as I was coming out of the anesthesia, the doctor came in and said, "Good news. You don't have Crohn's disease," as if he had saved the day. At this point, I think I'd been almost two months on the Ensure shakes and eating lots of smoothies and soft foods like mashed potatoes, noodles, and rice. My dad said to this man, "She still can't eat real food." The doctor said, "Well, if that works, okay for her. She should just keep doing that." My dad said, "No, I don't think you understand. She can't handle eating regular food; it hurts." He said, "Well, if she can eat the potatoes, then she can just eat the potatoes." Then he walked out of the room.

I remember one morning, I woke up, and I was shaking because I needed to eat. I grabbed some leftover cooked chicken out of the Tupperware in the fridge. I sat on that kitchen floor because that was as far as I could get, and my daughter sat next to me. That was our breakfast. We shared a piece of chicken that we ate with our fingers out of the Tupperware dish. I sat there until it digested a little bit, and I stopped shaking, and I thought, this is ridiculous. I can't even get her a proper breakfast, let alone make myself anything. What is wrong with me?

I don't know what the turning point was. Maybe it was lying on the couch for two weeks and not being able to eat normal food, and drinking soup broth, and not being able to take care of my daughter. I finally decided: I am not ninety-five. These are things that happen to someone who is at the end of her life. What is happening to me? Am I slowly dying off? I remember, growing up on the farm, we had a pony. His name was Peanut, and he was getting old. Ponies live longer than horses. If they live to be thirty, they have lived a good life. This one was thirty-six, and he was starting to get sick. I remember the vet came over. The pony had one problem here, another problem there. Things were just one on top of the other. The vet said, "Well, he is old, and his systems were structured to shut down. That is what happens when you get old."

I thought, my systems are starting to shut down.

Mary Beth Stutzman's systems were not shutting down. Something more fundamental was in play, a disease of civilization that each of us suffers from in one way or another. What ailed her was a specific condition brought on by the way we eat and live. But knowing some basics helps us understand how she got better (she did get better—dramatically better) and what this story means for each of us. We'll come back to her story soon enough.

CARBS TO SUGAR

The diseases that ail us, that list of burdens on our health and the leading causes of premature death and debilitation worldwide, can appear like a tangle of threads suggesting complexity. But if one simply recalls two fundamental and crucial facts— that these are diseases of civilization and that civilization is by definition the domestication and resulting dependence on grain agriculture—then the tangle is really a Gordian knot, ready to be cut with one big satisfying whack of the sword. There is actually a better name for the Gordian knot, and it is metabolic syndrome. This is medicine's name for a series of problems that run together like type 2 diabetes, heart disease, and obesity, all related to the metabolism of sugar.

If one reads the succession of diet books, one might come away with the incorrect impression that much of this problem remains unsettled. There are a couple of reasons for this confusion. First, over the course of researching evolutionary nutrition, science's ideas and assumptions about what our ancestors actually ate, the diet that made them so healthy, have changed, and some of that change is interesting. We have always looked to the past with a set of cultural blinders that allowed us to see what we wanted to see. This is unavoidable and only partially correctable, over time, by doing more science: picking through bones, sorting DNA and arrowheads. But the thing is, we will never know for sure; there will be blanks, and our cultural preconceptions, prejudices, and imaginations will fill in those blanks.

But there is a more unsettling factor in much of the disagreement and confusion. The dirty little secret of the whole business is that diet books sell well, and so it is often in the best interests of authors to argue that their prescription is very different — new and improved, to borrow a phrase from marketers — from preceding prescriptions. Interests of commerce dictate an emphasis on differences and disagreements. We think a better approach here is to cut back to fundamentals and begin on the common ground, and the common ground is the indisputable fact that for millions of years, our ancestors thrived on a diet that did not include dense packages of carbohydrates. They had a low-carb diet for the very simple reason (and also indisputable fact) that dense packages of carbohydrates for the most part did not exist. When you consider that these very same foods constitute something like 80 percent of all human nutrition today, you get some idea of the significance of this revolution. This is the correlation that counts: high consumption of carbohydrates with high incidence of disease related to carbohydrates. But we have more than a coincidence here. We can explain the mechanism by which it works.

The world of carbohydrates subdivides pretty endlessly, but the first cut is two classifications: complex and simple carbohydrates. The complex carbohydrates are more intricate molecules better known as starches, and this is the stuff of our main agricultural crops: corn, rice, wheat, and all grains, as well as potatoes. Fruits and vegetables do indeed contain carbohydrates, but in far smaller amounts, meaning they're far less concentrated. Starch from grains and potatoes is to spinach what a glass of 180 proof rum is to beer — and that's more than an analogy, because the same substance is in play. Alcohol comes from fermented, broken-down carbohydrates.

So where does sugar figure in? Simple. Sugars are the simple carbohydrates. You eat both complex and simple carbohydrates, but your digestion breaks both complex and simple into simple and simpler. The process of digestion of carbohydrates is a disassembly of the larger, complex molecules of starches to yield sugars, and this elemental and straightforward process begins in your mouth. So simple is the process that some starches are rendered into sugars through chewing and saliva even before they hit your throat. The result is a long list of sugars, but these in turn reduce to two in the main: glucose and fructose. For instance, table sugar or cane sugar, known as sucrose, is really about half glucose and half fructose, the latter so named because it is the dominant sugar in fruits. (And it's present in most fruits in laughably small amounts, compared with the sugar in, say, a glass of Coke, or even apple juice. That's the issue.)

The dominant industrial food process of our day is, in fact, simply a replication of this reduction, breaking down the starches of corn into sugars as high-fructose corn syrup. And even high-fructose corn syrup is, like sucrose, a combination of glucose and fructose: it's about 55 percent fructose, which is what the manufacturers mean by "high." Next time you hear an argument that somehow cane sugar is better than high-fructose corn syrup, bear in mind you are arguing about 50 percent versus 55 percent fructose.

But like one big, long funnel, this whole process, both natural digestion and factory manufacture, aims at a single point, which is glucose. Glucose is a fuel, the dominant fuel of our muscles and especially our brain, especially in today's sugar-saturated world. The glucose you eat as glucose goes straightaway to the bloodstream and, in theory, at least, goes to work. Fructose goes to your digestive system, and a couple of hours later, enzymes have converted it into glucose and sent it to your bloodstream.

But here is the dark little secret in all of this, and it sounds very odd to say it: glucose is toxic. It is poison, and the body regards it just that way. We have spent generations now in a search for toxins that sponsor the diseases that ail us, the industrial chemicals, pesticides, and pollutants that may kill us, and yes, these may be killing us. But the supreme irony in all of this is that the obvious toxin hides in plain sight. It's difficult to accuse the very substance on which all of civilization depends. People who consider these matters often refer to the "omnivore's dilemma," but it gets more and more difficult to claim to be omnivores, creatures that eat both plants and animals. The prima facie case is we have become carbovores as a result of our domestication by grain. This is the carbovore's dilemma: we exist for the most part on a substance that our bloodstream treats as a toxin.

Now wait a minute. Carbohydrates in food are nothing new, and hunter-gatherers ate them all along, even fairly dense packages as one might find in the tubers that were the precursors of domestic potatoes or in the wild grass seeds that were precursors of grain. Further, haven't we argued that the hallmark of the species is our adaptability, our nimbleness, our bodies' ability to adjust to novel conditions and balance its systems through homeostasis? So what if we are eating more concentrated forms of carbohydrates? That hardly qualifies as turning what was a basic food group for millions of years—and not just for humans but for the whole animal kingdom—into something we call toxic. Why don't our bodies simply adjust and head right back for homeostasis? The answer is, our bodies do.

Glucose is a very specific toxin, toxic in large doses *in the bloodstream*. This is precisely why the more extreme carbovores among us make a big deal about blood sugar level, the highs and lows that come with the balancing act—because it is a balancing act. And our bodies are highly adapted to execute this balancing act with a series of reactions all regulated by the hormone insulin. When glucose arrives in the bloodstream, it immediately and reliably (in everyone but those with type 1 diabetes) triggers the pancreas to secrete insulin, which sends a series of signals through the body, all with the central purpose of removing glucose from our bloodstream. Fast. Insulin oversees the body's response to toxicity. Glucose is a three-alarm fire that demands immediate reaction, which is why your brain pays so much attention to it—the blood sugar rush.

The body has basically two choices for getting glucose out of the bloodstream. The first and best answer is to send it off to muscles and organs, where it converts into a derivative called glycogen, a readily burnable fuel for our muscles. The catch is, the body has a very limited capacity for storing glycogen in muscle fibers—maybe enough energy to keep a marathon runner going for an hour or so, the quantity of glycogen from a few ounces of sugar. Further, unless you are a marathon runner, the majority of this storage space in muscles is already pretty full most of the time. So the body deals by going straight for plan B, which is to convert the glucose into fat and store it in ever broader bands around the stomach, butt, and thighs, depending on gender. (Gender determines which other hormones are present and where they are in the body to interact with insulin and guide the process of storing fat.)

There's a side chain to this process of fat conversion, again related to the fact that the body considers glucose to be toxic in the bloodstream and so makes its removal a priority. It is this: muscles burn glycogen to do work, but they are also capable of burning fat in parallel, both what we eat and what is stored. No need to convert back into glucose; fat itself burns very well to fuel muscles. We are told over and over again, especially in the world of athletics, that carbohydrates are your fuel. But the fine print, even in mainstream advice on this issue, reveals that fat is your fuel, too. And for endurance athletes especially, but even in day-to-day movement, fat is the most important fuel, or it is unless you have a surplus of glucose from eating too many carbohydrates. Back to insulin: remember, it is a hormone and so sends a variety of signals designed to remove glucose from your bloodstream. One of the strongest and clearest of those messages is to tell your body to stop burning fat and burn glucose instead as a priority. Coincident to this is a signal to stop moving fat from storage. The priority is to remove the glucose from the bloodstream.

None of this is a real problem, as long as one eats carbohydrates at levels at which we were evolved to eat them — that is, few and mixed with a variety of foods. This is our adaptability: the system is designed to return our bodies to homeostasis, a built-in regulator that makes glucose useful and keeps it out of the bloodstream at toxic levels. The problem arises when we overwhelm that system, when we deliver far more glucose and deliver it far more directly than our bodies were designed for.

Mode of delivery is as relevant as quantity. Remember that through most of human evolution, the majority of our carbohydrates came as the complex variety embedded in a matrix of fiber, which is to say foods. The digestion of this food took time, and so our bodies metered out the glucose in dribs and drabs through the course of a day. Now, though, we deliver many of our carbohydrates in the simple form, much of it as glucose, and sometimes not even in food at all but dissolved in water, a practice that completely bypasses the leveling effect of the digestive system. Sugar dissolved in water is the worst-case scenario, which is why soft drinks are so insidious and loom so large in the problem of childhood obesity around the world. But this is equally true of more socially accepted forms of dissolved sugar, such as fruit juices. That all-organic, all-natural fizzy fruit drink from the health-food store (no high-fructose corn syrup, only natural cane sugar) is every bit as damaging as a Coke, at least with respect to glucose. If you come away from this book with one rule and one rule only, it is this: don't drink sugar water. In any form. Not a Big Gulp Coke. Not a Knudsen's 100 percent natural and organic fruit juice.

But even in food and even in the form of complex carbohydrates such as the bagel you picked up this morning at Starbucks, the effect is only slightly less corrosive and sets you up for the crash, which is a condition called insulin resistance. It means that like those who repeatedly heard the boy who cried wolf, your body slowly becomes calloused to the constant ringing of the three-bell alarm of insulin. Your signals become crossed and this sends you eventually into the full-on crisis that is metabolic syndrome. This is the Gordian knot, the cluster of nasty little maladies that run together: obesity, heart disease, high blood pressure, type 2 diabetes, and stroke — and, less directly, cancer. Each of these is rooted in metabolic syndrome. This is the core of the emerging argument that sugar is toxic and sugar is responsible for what ails us. Carbs are responsible, too, because — as we've just shown — carbohydrates reduce to sugar.

The argument remains controversial, especially among nutritionists, or at least in the public pronouncements of nutritionists, and there is an issue embedded here that has more to do with the sociology of science than with the science itself. We have heard nutritionists acknowledge in private that fat is not the problem but turn around in public and say it is, simply because they are reluctant to abandon a fifty-year-old message. Doing so, they say, might confuse the public. The result, though, is a mixed set of messages, made even more mixed by the big-money politics of food and sugar and industrial agriculture — some of which is sinister, and some of which is simply wound up in bureaucratic inertia and human nature. The problem is, we have been told for a couple of generations that we are fat because we eat too much fat, and that's a much more direct argument and easier sell than saying—as we have here—that we are fat because we eat too much sugar and complex carbohydrates. Some of us do indeed eat too much fat, and we'll get to that in a moment, but first let's challenge the fat-o-phobes straight on. Fat is good for you, and we ought to stop saying otherwise.

THE RISE OF FAT-O-PHOBIA

The history of blaming fat for the cluster of diseases around metabolic syndrome, it turns out, is short and focused. Science has been thinking about obesity for at least a couple of centuries, but for only about fifty years have the arguments focused on fat. We can blame Ancel Keys and Dwight Eisenhower for this. Keys was a researcher at the University of Minnesota who was first known for a series of intriguing studies during World War II on the effects of starvation. He used conscientious objectors as the volunteers in his experiments and demonstrated that the psychological effects of starvation were extreme and included lifelong psychological debilitation, even after full nutrition returned. But he was better known for focusing on fat in general and cholesterol in particular. Keys is the reason most of us now know our cholesterol numbers.

Eisenhower's contribution to all of this was the heart attack he had while still serving as president, which greatly drew national attention to what was then, as now, a widespread health problem. And true enough, Eisenhower had by then given up his four-pack-a-day Camel habit, but he also had a high cholesterol number at about the time Keys, a messianic character, was trumpeting the evils of cholesterol to public health officials.

This case emerges in intriguing detail in the work of Gary Taubes, a science writer and historian. We recommend his book *Good Calories, Bad Calories*, which is far more comprehensive and important than the diet-book title might suggest. It is an exhaustive summary and builds a broad case about cholesterol, fat, and carbohydrates, but the story is best summarized by an old, peer-reviewed joke that Taubes uses and we repeat here. A guy walking down the street one night notices a drunk hunched over in a determined search under a lamppost. "What are you looking for?" "I lost my car keys." "Well, I'll help you look. Are you sure you dropped them here?" "Nah. I dropped 'em over there a ways, but the light's better over here."

The light that has focused our search on this matter for a couple of generations is the fact that doctors can easily measure cholesterol—which is one of hundreds of biochemicals vital to our system and yet somehow the one believed to reveal everything there is to know about heart disease. Cholesterol is technically a chemical form called a "lipid," a category that includes fats, but cholesterol itself is a sterol. It is nonetheless essential to every single cell in your body. But when we talk about cholesterol, we generally talk about lipoproteins, which are specialized structures the body makes to transport fats (including cholesterol) and proteins in the bloodstream. There are a variety of lipoproteins, and cholesterol is contained and freighted in each. There is no good way to measure cholesterol itself, so we measure lipoproteins as a proxy.

The first cut of classification gives us low-density lipoproteins (LDL) and high-density lipoproteins (HDL), the "bad" and "good" cholesterol, respectively. Those two and a third, triglycerides, make up the three common numbers of the garden-variety lipid profile. The focus is mostly on LDL, the so-called bad cholesterol. But not so fast. LDL itself subdivides into two distinct structures, according to size, and only the very small ones are thought to lead to damage. When your doctor uses your lipid profile to prescribe a lifetime of statin drugs and possibly a lifetime of the muscle cramping that is the known side effect, she often hasn't a clue which type of LDL particles dominate in your profile, despite evidence that says only one of these is associated with heart disease. Further, we have known about the two sizes of particles and their relative importance since cholesterol was first discovered early in the twentieth century, but mostly we ignore the distinction.

And further still, there is plenty of evidence that says heart disease is better predicted by triglyceride levels, and this number ramps up according to how much sugar you eat, not fat. And even further, a lipid profile that shows high triglycerides and low HDL is neatly predictive of the bad kind of LDL. This profile, and not high cholesterol or even high LDL, is far more strongly associated with heart disease.

The whole issue has become layered in misinformation and mythologies. For instance, there is the widespread belief that eating foods high in cholesterol will yield elevated cholesterol in your bloodstream. This is a straightforward enough assumption, but it's probably wrong. Taubes reviewed the evidence through the years and concluded, "Dietary cholesterol, for instance, has an insignificant effect on blood cholesterol. It *might* elevate cholesterol levels in a small percentage of highly sensitive individuals, but for most of us, it's clinically meaningless."

At the same time, a diet high in *carbohydrates* is strongly associated with high triglycerides, low HDL, and the damaging particles of LDL, which is the killer profile. And none of this is new, although it has been borne out by new studies. Even before Keys began his mission, there was plenty of evidence to contradict his views. A whole generation of nutritionists have rested arguments on Keys's famous Seven Countries Study, a piece of work he said proved his hypothesis about the connection between dietary fat and heart disease. The problem is, Keys analyzed data from twenty-two countries and deliberately assembled a list of the first seven that made his point and ignored the longer list of countries that contradicted it.

The irony here is that the misguided attack on all fats and cholesterol targeted high-cholesterol foods like eggs and butter and argued that we would be better off eating highly processed substitutes like Egg Beaters and margarine. Which brings us to the fats, and the refinement of the argument about fats. Those substitutes had in common a type of fat that is manufactured and has no precedent in evolutionary history: what we call "trans fats," which is a truncation of their technical chemical name, trans-isomer fatty acids. These are also labeled "unsaturated fats," but the better way to think of them is as not existing in nature. These are the fats that harm you, and together with sugar they are the foundation of the industrial foods system.

The damage began with Crisco. Procter & Gamble used a process called hydrogenization—a way to turn oils into solid fats—to invent and introduce Crisco, billed as a lard substitute, in 1911. The same process has since spawned a string of fat substitutes, all based in vegetable oil—especially oil that derives from processing corn and soybeans. It was, for the food industry, a way to spin what was then a waste product of our farm surplus production into a marketable product, and marketing was the key. The early campaigns to sell the public on shortening and margarine were the prototypes for today's sea of hype and cynicism that is the processed foods system. These are the roots of fast food.

The problem with trans fats is that hydrogenation created a set of fatty acid molecules unprecedented in our digestive systems. We are not evolved to handle them. As often as not, foreign molecules in the body rightly trigger an immune response, including inflammation. Inflammation, in turn, is every bit as important as, if not more important than, cholesterol in the genesis of arteriosclerosis and the resulting heart disease. That is, there is a pretty direct and logical link between heart disease and the margarine once marketed as the heart-healthy substitute for butter. By the 1950s, nutritionists were beginning to suspect that link. Epidemiologists now estimate that every 2 percent increase in consumption of trans fats increases the collective risk of heart disease by 23 percent. The National Academy of Sciences says that no level of trans fats in our food is safe. None. Because they are so tied up with heart disease, this, of course, strikes straight at the core of one of our most important diseases of civilization—but there are also linkages here that one might not expect. For instance, a study in 2011 showed that eating trans fats greatly increases the risk of clinical depression, which—as you will recall—is identified as a rapidly growing problem worldwide and, we argue, a disease of civilization.

In the case of trans fats, a measured dose of fat-o-phobia may well be in order, and one should avoid them like the plague. Unfortunately, the bad advice on other fats that began with Ancel

Keys tarred some of our healthiest foods with the same brush, and this needs to be corrected, especially in the case of omega-3s. That's a term you have heard and may well have heard in nutritional advice like this. Step one: Avoid fats. Step two: Be sure to get a good supply of omega-3s. This is not so much advice as it is a hangover of fat-o-phobia. Omega-3s are fats—fats that are in critically short supply in our diets. This shortage may well be a factor in widespread depression but also in high cholesterol, heart disease, inflammation, and compromised brain development.

The clue to the importance of all of this is the name of the category that includes omega-3s, which is essential fatty acids. They are labeled "essential" because without them we could not survive. Literally. We get omega-3s from a variety of sources, but mostly from free-range meats, especially cold-water fish. Vegetarians get them from the few plant sources that contain them, such as walnuts or flax oil.

Their counterparts are omega-6 fats, also present in meat, and although omega-6s are seeing some bad press lately, they are also essential fatty acids. The problem is one of balance—and again, this is rooted in our industrial system of agriculture. Cows evolved to eat grass, but mostly we no longer feed them grass; we feed them the corn and soybeans that are the prime products of our industrial agriculture system. The practice creates beef high in omega-6 fats and low in omega-3s. The practice of fattening beef in feedlots and the preponderance of factory beef in the fast-food system passes this omega-3 shortage into our bodies.

But this is also why eating red meat itself has gotten a bad rap, with endless strings of studies linking it to heart disease and a variety of other issues. The beef that is the basis of these conclusions is factory beef, and no wonder.

Meanwhile, the shortage of omega-3s undoubtedly shows up in areas we might not suspect, and one example from the literature demonstrates just how far-reaching this effect might be. One researcher in education—not in nutrition—performed a meta-analysis of all peer-reviewed research on proven methods to increase a child's intelligence (that is, boost academic performance). The conclusion: "Supplementing infants with long-chain polyunsaturated fatty acids [specifically omega-3s], enrolling children in early educational interventions, reading to children in an interactive manner, and sending children to preschool all raise the intelligence of young children."

(We think there is enough evidence to add exercise to the list, but the point stands.)

And it is a problem that can be easily solved by eating grass-finished beef, now widely available thanks to increased awareness and demand, but also wild-caught fish, free-range eggs, and even walnuts. This is a corrective to generations' worth of bad assumptions about fats. And yes, our bloodstreams are full of fat as a result of the industrial diet and processed food, but this is not all fat's fault. Remember the insulin response and the insulin resistance generated by excess carbohydrate consumption. Remember that insulin immediately shuts off the body's use of fat; it sends signals to keep it in storage and at the same time signals muscles to cease burning fat and start burning glucose. This alone goes a long way toward explaining why fatty acids jam up in our bloodstream, especially as triglycerides. It's not because we are eating fats; people always have. It is because excessive carbohydrates, especially sugar, are preventing us from burning them. Cut out the carbs, and the fat problem takes care of itself, as long as you eat the right kinds of fats.

But in his book, Taubes takes on this issue from another direction, a convincing capstone of an argument. There is no doubt that obesity is increasing in a number of countries around the world. In the United States, we can plot that increase on a graph over the last fifty or so years. And we can plot, alongside that, three other graphs, for per capita consumption of protein, fats, and carbohydrates (including sugars). The first two graphs show flat lines with no real increase in per capita consumption of either protein or fats. In sharp distinction, per capita consumption of carbohydrates in the United States has risen steadily in marked and obvious parallel to obesity.

This is not a new trend. Annual per capita sugar consumption in the United States was 5 pounds per person in 1700, 23 pounds in 1800, 70 pounds in 1900, and 152 pounds today. This is why we talk about sugar when we begin talking about what ails us. Want to go wild? Here's how. Don't eat sugar, not in any form. Not sucrose, not pure cane sugar, not high-fructose corn syrup, not honey, not in all those other polysyllabic chemical names that reveal industrial processes rooted in corn: maltodextrin, dextrose, sorbitol, mannitol. Not apple juice. John thinks this is one of the hidden causes of childhood obesity, even in households where there is very good parenting.

Don't eat dense packages of carbohydrates, particularly refined flour. No bread, no pasta, no bagels, certainly no cookies. No grain, period, not even whole grain. Don't eat trans fats. Period. And you may have figured out the derivative rule by now. Trans fats and sugars are the foundation of processed food. Do not eat processed food.

You will notice that in this prescription, we have remained silent on the topic of dairy products, and not because the topic is irrelevant. Dairy is, in fact, interesting both for what it tells us about evolution and also in the ways it resonates through your health and well-being.

To begin with, dairy is one of the more outstanding—if not *the* outstanding—exceptions to the rule that the basic human design has not changed in fifty thousand years. The fact is, about a third of humanity has evolved the ability to digest lactose, the sugar in milk, as adults. All children make the enzyme lactase (the gene product that digests lactose) for the obvious reason that baby mammals have to digest milk to survive. But in deep evolutionary time, all adults lost that ability as we matured, which was not a problem in our ancestral homeland in Africa, near the equator, with ample sunlight. But as humans migrated north, winters brought shorter days, less sun, and a vitamin D deficiency, which was a serious problem. (And as we shall see, it still is a serious problem.) We get vitamin D from the sun, but also from milk.

In evolution, necessity does indeed mother invention, and it was in Eurasia that a mutation occurred that allowed adults to digest lactose. To this day, that ability tracks in populations with roots in Eurasia, the third of us who can tolerate lactose into adulthood.

But interestingly, there was a parallel step in cultural, not biological, evolution that solved the same problem. Around the Mediterranean and on the Asian steppes, there is widespread lactose intolerance in the populations, yet these people eat dairy products like cheeses and yogurt and have for a very long time. They have adopted a cultural practice that outsources the job of digesting lactose: fermentation. Fermentation uses bacteria to digest lactose, meaning that people with lactose intolerance can still get nutrition and vitamin D from fermented dairy products. They are using an external microbiome, an ingenious bit of outsourcing.

We have remained silent on dairy in our prescription because this evolutionary history outlines some individual solutions. Do what works for you.

WHY VARIETY

Close readers will notice by now that our argument appears to have painted us into a corner, and it is precisely the same predicament that traps most diet nags, an argument that we become ill and fat by eating this or that food. Because we are not just talking about quantity here; we are talking about restricting a whole class of foods, and humanity's most important foods at that. This contention runs smack up against the evolutionary foundation of humanity that we laid out in the beginning: we humans are the ultimate generalists, the Swiss Army knives of not just movement but nutrition, too. The foundation of our success as a species is our ability to adapt to a wide range of conditions, environments, and foods—the very ability that allowed us to occupy the entire planet, unlike any other species. In fact, we are not going to shy away from this apparent contradiction. Not only did evolution equip us so we can eat a wide variety of foods, but it made variety a necessary condition of our well-being. We not only can but must have variety to be healthy. Remember, this was George Armelagos's second and more important rule, a fact so often missed in books that attempt to adapt evolutionary understanding to prescriptions.

"I think variety is the key to all of it," he says.

Even our argument that you should not eat sugar does not violate this rule; restricting sugar enables the body's responses that support variety. Remember homeostasis, the complex array of thermostats that allow our bodies to roll with the punches? Homeostasis underscores much of what we have to say. These thermostats let us weather variation and return to a sustainable state. Insulin's response to sugar in the bloodstream is homeostasis at work. But insulin resistance is the signal that we have swamped that system, so much so that our internal thermostats cease to function and therefore cease to enable us to navigate the world of diversity and variety.

This is the negative side of the argument, and the positive side is more intriguing still. The enormous energetic demands of our brains mean, as we have seen, that we could not be at all casual about nutrition. The demand for energetically dense foods dictated that we eat meat, which meant hunting, which in turn required a great deal of intelligence. But it also meant gathering plants, which in turn required detailed knowledge of plants, seasons, and even subtle clues like what sort of leaf pattern in what sort of state of wilt signaled that a succulent tuber was hidden a few feet under the ground, ready for harvest. Our attention to color, our empathy for animals, our recognition of patterns, even our ability to communicate with one another—all are rooted in this fundamental need to feed our brains, and at the same time, our brains return the favor by allowing it all, a sort of positive feedback loop that drives development. We revel in all of this and take pleasure in it, still enjoying a primal rush of pleasure on walking through a bustling farmer's market on a sunny afternoon.

But the whole array of demands gets ratcheted up to another

level still when we add to this what has come to be called the omnivore's dilemma, a dilemma caused by conflicting interests. Because we are omnivores and because we range over the entire planet, it is in our interests to exploit as many food sources as possible. This means that an important characteristic of omnivores is bred to the bone in humans: we are neophiliacs. We have to be. We have an innate love of novelty, of variety, a need to sample new things. And at the same time, some of those bright and shiny new things, some of those foods on offer in the wild, are poisonous—a lot more than you might think. Not acutely so, like sugar, but lethal poisons that drop you dead on the spot. Thus, it is equally in our interests to be neophobes, to fear new things, thereby causing a conflict at the center of the human condition.

Throughout the course of our evolutionary history, we have negotiated this dilemma with cuisine, sharing cultural information about what is good to eat and not good to eat. We depend on others—elders, mothers, and fathers—to hold this information specific to place and teach it to those who need it. It is the very essence of culture, one more way in which we depend on one another for survival. And there is nothing perfect about this solution; if it were perfect, a given culture long adapted to a given place would make use of all the nutritious plants and animals and leave all the poisonous ones alone. Not the case. For instance, in one of his papers on this topic, Armelagos reports that the !Kung people of the Kalahari Desert eat a total of 105 species of plants and 260 species of animals from the desert savanna environment—a total of 365 species of plants and animals. But modern biologists have determined that the same place holds at least 500 edible species. The gap is a measure of the cultural negotiation of the omnivore's dilemma on the safe side. Still, the undeniable push in humanity is toward variety.

Tyler Graham and Drew Ramsey are not evolutionary biologists but a science writer and a medical doctor, respectively, and their argument, summarized in their book *The Happiness Diet*, does not derive from !Kung practices but from modern humans. They argue as we do that our happiness and mental well-being are rooted in what we eat, and this is more than a matter of depression. For instance, trace brain-derived neurotrophic factor, or BDNF. In *Spark*, John called this chemical "Miracle-Gro for the brain." It is the important link that explains why simple exercise can have such a profound effect on cognition and well-being, and we'll have more to say about it in the next chapter, when we address movement. But nutrition affects BDNF, too. Eating a diet high in sugar decreases BDNF. Eating foods with folate, vitamin B12, and omega-3 fats increases BDNF in the brain, just as exercise does.

Graham and Ramsey examine a list of twelve micronutrients and vitamins: vitamin B12, iodine, magnesium, cholesterol, vitamin D, calcium, fiber, folate, vitamin A, omega-3s, vitamin E, and iron; each is plentiful in the very foods, like fresh fruits and vegetables, that we have eliminated from the modern industrial diet, and each is vital to brain health and well-being on very specific pathways. But this is just the beginning. We are starting to understand the phenomenon of bioavailability, which says that addressing the lack of a given vitamin or micronutrient is not simply a matter of adding a given amount back through a supplement. The body's ability to absorb those nutrients is greatly influenced by the presence or absence of other nutrients. For instance, eating spinach with lemon helps the body absorb much more of the iron in the spinach. Eating eggs and cheese together delivers a better uptake of vitamin D and calcium.

What emerges is the rough outline of a picture far too complex to detail in a prescriptive diet, and in the end, that's the point. Yes, we can keep track of some of this in the cultural wisdom that has evolved through the millennia, but in the end, we're simply not able, as individuals, to account for all of it, to count the calories, read the labels, and total the RDAs for a long list of necessary nutrients. The case that emerges, then, is precisely the situation evolution prepared us for. We can only begin to satisfy the complex and highly evolved requirements of our bodies, especially our brains, through variety. That's why evolution hard-wired us to value it so greatly.

And the fact is, no one understands this fundamental, innate drive for variety more than the modern-day marketers of industrial and processed food. Walk through the aisle of any convenience store or thumb through ads for fast-food chains, soft drinks, and box cereals. Note the variety, exotic names, every shape, color, and texture imaginable. This is what we crave. Then begin reading labels and note the predominance of the suffixes "-trose" and "-crose," i.e., sugar, and of corn and corn derivatives, processed soybeans, trans fats, and flour. The variety is an illusion. Under the label and chemical colorings and aromas, it is the same deadly industrial blend.

All of this forms the outline of our prescription, and the first half we've already given you is indeed negative: to not eat sugar, dense carbohydrates like grains, and trans fats, which is to say processed foods. But this is really advice to reject the monotony of the modern industrial diet. We are not urging a diet or even calorie restriction; we are outlining a sustainable way of life, and it rests on variety: the profusion and explosion of flavors, colors, and textures that evolution tuned our senses to pursue. Nuts, root vegetables, leafy greens, fruits, fish, wild game, clean, cool water. Range far and wide. Eat well.

BACK TO MARY BETH STUTZMAN

We caught up again with Mary Beth Stutzman during a quiet summer's evening in 2013 over dinner in a pleasant little restaurant at the mouth of northern Michigan's Thunder Bay River. She was well. We ordered, and she decided to pass on the local lake-caught fish fillets, which on the surface may seem a bit odd, because she is an active booster of the local sport fishery and even has her own television show dedicated to the topic. It's how she supports her community, and that's part of what she is about and glad to do now that she is well.

But the restaurant's fillets came breaded. No bread—no way. That's the rule that made her well. That was the key she was looking for in all those years of traipsing to specialists and emergency rooms doubled over in pain. She found the solution not from any advice from an MD but by accident. Just about the time she thought she was going to die, a friend happened to bring her some cupcakes to cheer her up. The irony is, the friend himself knew better than to eat cupcakes, but he thought Mary Beth might like them. He also brought her a book on the paleo diet, which he himself had adopted and which was why he didn't eat cupcakes. She read the book, particularly the section about a problem called leaky gut, which sounded terribly, achingly, shockingly familiar. Leaky gut is caused by eating dense, refined carbs and sugar. In all those years of seeing doctors and delivering long lists of symptoms, no one suggested this to her, let alone asked what she was eating. No one asked about her nutrition. She adopted the diet and got immediately and noticeably better. And better. And better. Food healed her. It's as simple as that.

Now she is vibrant and alive, an exercise enthusiast, actively promoting fitness as fun. She is engaged with her family and happy.

"I can't even describe how great I felt. It was like being born again. It was a feeling of how great it is to be alive. It was out of this world," she told us.

And no, she is not a food fanatic; in fact, she loathes the term "paleo." If you press her on this matter, she'll simply label her diet "trending toward paleo." She even allows herself occasional tastes of selected whole grains, and now and again a little ice cream with its sugar. She's okay with a little lactose. And maybe this variation and experimentation, even more than her diet and recovery, are the lessons we'd like you to carry with you as we develop our story. Here, though, are some key points: First, her path to well-being began with diet, specifically with recognizing the basic fact that civilization's grain and sugar were making her ill, and even—as a young woman—close to death. All she had to do to fix it was pay some reasonable attention to diet—nothing extreme, but simply head in the direction of eating the way humans were evolved to eat. Second, she used that knowledge to devise her own path through the pitfalls. But most important, once she started to get better, her path to well-being led beyond diet, through other areas like fitness, family, and community. You will see this happen to others as we go on. Not every pathway begins with diet and nutrition, although many do, and it's hard to imagine getting better if nutrition is wrong. But in some way or another, we think every pathway begins with a lesson from evolution.

CAUTION: EVOLUTION RUNS BOTH WAYS

There is a popular myth about evolution: that it is progressive and leads only one way, to bigger, better, and smarter, to more complex. It can lead that way, because complexity takes time to assemble, so complex comes later. But so does simpler, and the koala bear, that cuddly icon of cute, is our favorite example. Koalas are interesting to biologists because they eat only one thing, eucalyptus leaves, so they inhabit these trees ubiquitous in Australia. As a result, they really never have to leave the trees; they can just sit and watch the world go by, day in, day out.

It wasn't always so. Koalas once had a more diverse diet in their evolutionary history. The mark of this is inside their head, as their brain does not fill the entire space allotted for it in their skull. That's because, coincident with adopting the narrower diet, their brain shrank, and evolution has not yet had time to make skull size compensate, so the tiny little brain rattles around in a too-big case. One single source of food. That, and they are sedentary. If the koalas wanted to retain the bigger brain that evolution gave them, they also needed to move, and this is the lesson we turn to next.

4

Nimble

*Building and Rebuilding the
Brain Through Movement*

No one can be blamed for being confused about this matter, particularly those who follow health news in the popular press. Dueling headlines appear almost daily summarizing the latest published results and fronting pronouncements such as this one from a recent paragraph in the *New York Times*' health section: "And in a just world, frequent physical activity should make us slim. But repeated studies have shown that many people who begin an exercise program lose little or no weight. Some gain."

The fact is, we don't care whether the studies like the ones reported here are the final word on the matter. (We don't think they are.) The larger issue is far more important: these sorts of conclusions are irrelevant. Physical exercise is not about weight loss; it is about your well-being.

The British scientist Daniel Wolpert likes to begin his case with the sort of fundamental and vexing question that seriously shakes up our thinking: why do we have a brain? He expects the obvious answer: to think.

"But this is completely wrong," he says. "We have a brain for one reason only: to produce adaptable and complex movements. There is no other plausible explanation." He is saying that our brains are literally built on and inextricably tied to movement of our bodies. Movement builds our brain because movement requires a brain.

Wolpert's career of researching this traces the same argument that people often use about basic intelligence: that computers can't do what we do. After generations of trying, the best and brightest of computer science still have been unable to approach something like artificial intelligence, and what we mean by that is that we can't program computers to perform music, exercise judgment, or write books. Wolpert thinks something is missing in this familiar argument: "While computers can now beat grand masters at chess, no computer can yet control a robot to manipulate a chess piece with the dexterity of a six-year-old child."

This is because even the simplest of motions—a flick of a finger or a turn of the hand to pick up a pencil—is maddeningly complex and requires coordination and computational power beyond electronic abilities. For this you need a brain. One of our favorite quotes on this matter comes from the neuroscientist Rodolfo Llinás: "That which we call thinking is the evolutionary internalization of movement."

The telling encapsulation of this argument is the case of the sea squirt, a primitive sea animal with a rudimentary nervous system. For part of its life, the squirt spends time moving but only to look for a spot where it can anchor itself in the path of a ready source of food. On doing so, its first act is to eat and digest its own brain; it doesn't need one anymore because it no longer needs to move.

Yet this is the sort of linkage between brain and movement that holds up from sea squirt to human along the long evolutionary chain. The association is clear: the more a species needs to move, the bigger its brain—a relationship particularly pronounced in mammals. And although we don't often think of it this way, the argument gets its clincher with the great ape that (a) has the very largest of brains (we humans) and (b) happens to be the champion of movement. Coincidence, you think? One of our greatest and enduring fascinations as humans is with movement. Sedentary as we may be, we still pay enormous amounts of money and invest enormous amounts of cultural capital in watching people move, obviously so with sports but consider, too, movement like ballet. What other species could accomplish this level of variation and control in pure movement? Our attraction to ballet and dance is not coincidence, just as our deep appreciation for a naked human body of the gender that attracts us is not coincidence. This attraction is evolution's way of making us pay attention to what matters, and movement matters. Evolution has made us think that graceful movement is beautiful.

BRAIN BUILDING

Neuroscience in the '90s delivered a game-changing set of realizations that shone a couple of bright lights in new directions on the concepts of neuroplasticity and neurogenesis. The first says your brain is plastic in the prechemical sense of the word, malleable, shape-shifting, moldable. It is not the hardwired, compartmentalized organ we once thought it to be; it's not true that given cells and networks of cells and given areas and structures of the brain are assigned a task and that's that. Lose a set of cells to, say, a stroke, and you lose the ability to perform that task. Or, more to the point, get dealt a weak spot by genetics, say for language, and you will always have a struggle with language. But the brain can, in fact, rewire itself, repurpose bits and pieces. It can adapt. It grows. This is neuroplasticity.

Neurogenesis says something similar but even more revolutionary. New cells and networks of the brain grow as needed, very much as muscles grow with exercise. In fact, new-era neuroscience says that the brain is a muscle. This is more than an analogy. As science began to understand these phenomena, it began to tease out mechanisms, the cascades of signals and biochemicals that triggered this exquisite set of responses. This line of inquiry greatly illuminated what evolutionary biologists had already realized: that big brains and intricate physical movement went together, that evolution had in fact used some of the same principles to signal brain growth that it had used to signal muscle growth. Through time, evolution used biochemistry to enhance muscles, movement, and brains.

So far in our story, we have relied often on the concept of homeostasis, which is an array of signaling mechanisms within the body that responds to shocks or changes in the environment to return systems to a normal operating state. We'll see it again and again to the point of ramping up to a new level of complexity and a new idea as our argument develops. All in time. But at this point in the discussion we need another related idea: hormesis. Hormesis is a biological response to low doses of a stressor, such as a toxin, that improves the ability of the body to handle that toxin. It can be applied to exercise. Unlike homeostasis, hormesis does not return the body to a normal state. It returns it to a better-than-normal state. When a bodybuilder lifts weights, he is placing heavy stress on a given set of muscles, a process that damages them by overload. The body reacts with an immune response and inflammation. And now notice that we have introduced two troubling words into the discussion, at least troubling in terms of the popular understanding: inflammation and stress. The fact is, the body uses both to rebuild, and we'll argue later for a more refined appreciation of these forces.

But for now, the important point is that rebuilding the body does not simply build back what was torn down: it builds bigger and better, an adaptive response. Your muscles face a new challenge in the form of heavier weights, so the body responds by building infrastructure to meet that challenge. It grows and makes the body more resilient. Take the challenge away, and the body heads in the other direction: once again, use it or lose it.

And now we come back to BDNF, brain-derived neurotrophic factor, the Miracle-Gro of the brain. Movement places demands on the brain, just as it does on muscle, and so the brain releases BDNF, which triggers the growth of cells to meet the increased mental demands of movement. But BDNF floods throughout the brain, not just to the parts engaged in movement. Thus, the whole brain flourishes as a result of movement. It provides the environment that brain cells need to grow and function well.

Chemically, there is more to this story—lots more. For instance, exercise also triggers responses in the important neurotransmitters long studied in connection with issues like addiction and depression, chemicals like serotonin, dopamine, and norepinephrine. These are parallel processes. It all hangs together. But in the end, cells are cells. The brain is an energy-burning network of specially adapted cells like any other organ and is wrapped up in the health of the rest of the system. This ought to follow logically from the connection between the brain and movement: if the body needs stronger or more refined movement to meet a given challenge, it will need more brain circuitry to guide that movement. It would make no sense adaptively to build one without the other, so we need the biochemical provisions to do both.

This is no longer conjecture or theoretical construct. We may be a sedentary culture, but while we've been couch-bound in front of video games and computer monitors, science has been busy assembling a massive pile of evidence that says the quickest, surest path to the health and well-being of the brain and body is movement, or vigorous aerobic exercise.

Begin by considering a formal review of the literature, now more than a decade old but with conclusions that have even more support today. Writing in the *Journal of Applied Physiology*, researchers including Frank W. Booth laid out the case that inactivity was a looming factor in at least twenty "of the most chronic disorders." Yes, it does include obesity, but it extends far beyond to other afflictions of civilization, including congestive heart failure, coronary artery disease, angina and myocardial infarction, hypertension, stroke, type 2 diabetes, dyslipidemia, gallstones, breast cancer, colon cancer, prostate cancer, pancreatic cancer, asthma, chronic obstructive pulmonary disease, immune dysfunction, osteoarthritis, rheumatoid arthritis, osteoporosis, and a range of neurological dysfunctions, a subcategory of particular interest here and one we will unpack in a moment.

In almost all of these cases, the causes of the disease are directly linked to inactivity, but not all. For instance, Booth concludes that there is no evidence saying inactivity *causes* chronic obstructive pulmonary disease. That is, exercise may not prevent it but can heal it once it does occur—an important distinction. This is the realization that ought to ring through public discourse like a loud pealing bell, given that the list cited above is hugely responsible for the crushing burden of health-care costs in our society—and yet almost nowhere in the widespread discussion of reducing those costs do we mention how much of that bill is traceable to our sedentary ways.

In Booth's analysis of all of this, there is a simple sentence that greatly adds to the urgency. We are not just talking about sick people or physical debilitation. He writes: "Sedentary lifestyle is associated with lower cognitive skills." Stated more bluntly still, our inactivity is making us dumber. If anything, this conclusion can now be stated even more confidently, given the wealth of research in the decade since Booth made it. Both epidemiology and neuroscience have described the biochemistry that makes it so.

The definitive statement about this comes from a group of researchers headed by J. Eric Ahlskog from the Department of Neurology at the Mayo Clinic. Prompted by some inconclusive work by the National Institutes of Health, Ahlskog and his group undertook a comprehensive review of all the research they could find on the relationship between cognition and exercise. They used the keywords "cognition" and "exercise" to search the massive PubMed database of medical research. The search returned 1,603 published research papers on the topic, a number that in itself gives us some idea of how thoroughly this issue has been examined. And the researchers read every one of those papers and compiled conclusions in a paper of their own published in 2011.

Their emphasis was on dementia, in its severe form as Alzheimer's disease but also as evidenced in problems like the memory loss and decline of mental acuity that we think of as a sign of aging. Their results are sweeping and speak to all of us, not just the elderly. First, the preponderance of those 1,603 studies showed that exercise delivered marked improvements for people suffering all the cognitive impairments examined, from minor memory loss to full-on Alzheimer's. Further, the studies that examined middle-aged people who exercised regularly found a substantial preventive effect of all forms of impairment later in life. Exercise helps the afflicted but also prevents the affliction. Cognitive impairment is not so much a consequence of aging as it is a consequence of our sedentary lives.

Yet the consequences of dementia in our society are huge and getting much worse. A 2013 study by the Rand Corporation showed that now about 15 percent of people older than 71 — 3.8 million people — suffer from dementia. But the aging of baby boomers along with the way we live will nearly triple that number by 2040, to 9.1 million people. In addition, another 5.4 million people, 22 percent of those older than 71, suffer mild cognitive impairment, as opposed to full-on dementia. Current social costs of treating dementia alone in the United States are $109 billion, more than we spend treating either heart disease or cancer.

One might think the reason for this decline during old age is obvious. We have long thought that many of the late-life neuro-logical problems of aging stem directly from the decline of the cardiovascular system, that poor circulation robs the brain of oxygen. The group at the Mayo Clinic did indeed follow this trail and did indeed find what they called a "vascular" effect. But interestingly, the weight of the evidence caused them to con-clude this was secondary. The main benefit of exercise, they wrote, was improved neuroplasticity and neurogenesis. Specifi-cally, they traced this to the key neurotrophic factors of exercise, the Miracle-Gro effect with BDNF that we have talked about, but also to a group of parallel biochemicals, especially IGF-1, or insulin-like growth factor.

To take this line of reasoning one step further, the research-ers were able to find a number of papers in the pool that looked at brain growth—actual, physical, measurable brain growth—as a result of exercise and found that seniors who exercised devel-oped "significantly larger hippocampal volumes," and because the hippocampus participates in memory processing, they had improved memory as a result. They found that exercise also pre-vented a loss of gray matter overall (a loss common in aging) and, additionally, improved brain function as measured by func-tional magnetic resonance imaging, showing better and more robust connections throughout.

But now consider the word "aging," which doesn't just refer to old people. We are all aging, and as is the case with gravity on the rest of our bodies, the downward forces on our brains begin early and extend through life. This research is therefore relevant to all of life. We may well notice the loss of memory at age seventy-one, but it began a lot earlier. Which means there is every reason to start looking at this issue at the other end of life.

ALL EDUCATION IS PHYSICAL EDUCATION

There is an emerging and every-bit-as-robust body of research on the effects of exercise on young brains. Maybe the best example is not a research paper (although the project certainly has spawned its share of publications) but the long-running educational experiment that was the centerpiece of John Ratey's book *Spark*. If you haven't read the details of that case or the rest of the evidence presented in *Spark*, it's worth doing so to see this issue unfold. But we can encapsulate it here by citing the experiment in the Naperville school district, which demonstrates unequivocally how exercise builds brains at the beginning of life. The Naperville school district became the national leader in recognizing this by integrating a comprehensive program of aerobic workouts into the daily routine for its students. The program has paid off handsomely in stunning improvements in academic performance, improvement at the level that would in and of itself benchmark the sort of education reform that the nation needs and never seems able to accomplish.

But as is the case with research on aging, the body of evidence regarding exercise has only grown since. To date, no one we know of has gone so far as to compile in meta-analysis all the research on exercise and young people, as was done with the Mayo Clinic study. Nonetheless, there are some large and compelling data sets that prove the point. One of our favorites is a result in California, where state officials looked at eight hundred thousand fifth-, seventh-, and ninth-grade students, ranking their performance on a series of six physical fitness standards against their scores on standardized math and language tests.

The result was a clean, stair-stepped relationship: the more fitness standards a student met, the better the test scores.

Meanwhile, Sweden has assembled a massive database looking at 1.2 million boys who entered military service between 1950 and 1976, measuring both cardiovascular fitness and muscle strength against IQ and cognitive abilities when all the subjects were fifteen years old and again at eighteen. Cardiovascular fitness did indeed demonstrate the same positive relationship with both intellectual measurements. This study, however, went further and tracked the subjects into adulthood, finding that those with better fitness scores wound up with better education, more life satisfaction, and higher socioeconomic standing.

But there is an even more intriguing pattern in the Swedish case. The data set included 270,000 brothers and 1,300 identical twins and showed that cardio fitness and not familial relationship turned out to be the better predictor of both cognitive ability and IQ. That is, despite the popular assumption that IQ is genetically determined, fitness and not genes held the greater sway over these tests of intellect.

All of this traces to a thread of this idea that John has been following since the 1970s, when he first noticed that marathon runners suffered depression when they quit running. Stopping running was like stopping effective medication. This phenomenon goes beyond cognition to tie in the element of mental health.

Lately, and since John detailed these issues in *Spark*, there continues to be an ever-widening use of exercise in treating mental issues. We are seeing paper after paper showing positive results in treating anxiety, addictions, attention deficit disorder, obsessive-compulsive disorder, schizophrenia, and, lately, bipolar disorder, but nowhere has there been as much work done as with depression. In 2010, the American Psychiatric Association issued new guidelines for treating depression, and for the first time, exercise was listed as a proven treatment. Thus, the APA finally caught up with Hippocrates, who recommended that all people in a bad mood should go for a walk—and if it did not improve, walk again. The APA's change of heart was fostered by a lot of this convincing new evidence.

Psychologist James Blumenthal of Duke University has been leading the charge. He conducted trials looking at the effects of exercise on sedentary patients with anxiety or depression, and his research culminated in a seminal report in 1999. In this study, 156 sedentary depressed patients were assigned to one of three groups. One used increasing doses of sertraline, or Zoloft (a popular antidepressant), another began exercising three times a week for forty minutes each day, and the third received both the drug and the exercise regimen. At sixteen weeks there was no difference in their depression scores, but at the end of a ten-month follow-up, those still exercising were better off than those on pills alone.

Blumenthal was criticized by prominent psychopharmacologists for not having a placebo group, and so he completed another study, published in 2007, with 202 patients, showing similar positive results for those doing exercise. Since then there have been many other studies looking at both aerobic exercise and strength training, and both interventions show positive effects. Movement regimens such as yoga and tai chi also help, but not as much.

But looking at this impressive body of evidence—evidence largely absent in the public discussion of issues like education and health care—it's easy enough to miss the most significant accomplishment of the research. The evidence begins with what we will call the epidemiological case, that is, a statistical examination of outcomes for people who exercise. This can take us only so far; it steers us toward the pitfall that scientists understand when they warn us that correlation is not cause. This is the very pitfall that allowed, say, tobacco companies to wriggle out of responsibility when early epidemiological studies showed that smoking was associated with lung cancer. But years later, science was able to delineate and prove the biochemical linkages that made this so. They described *how* smoking caused lung cancer, and now there is no doubt. Not many people have noticed, but we are well past that point now with brain health and exercise. Sedentary behavior causes brain impairment, and we know how: by depriving your brain of the flood of neurochemistry that evolution developed in order to grow brains and keep them healthy.

WILD MOTION

So we've made the case and now you see the next step coming, the directive to pay up the gym membership, squeeze into the Lycra, load yourself onto a treadmill or stationary bike six days a week, set the timer for thirty minutes, punch up the iPod workout playlist, and slog your way to health. You know the drill, but if you think this is it, then you haven't been paying attention. The regimen described above is to movement what processed fast food is to a full-on feast. The gym drill may get you by—and we're not against it—but this is about going wild, about getting better, being as good as you can be. There is a better way to move.

We hope to entice you out of the gym and, toward that end, invite you on a run with us, a late spring day of the sort that pulls you outdoors, the first day this year without gloves and a jacket, cold at first, but sun and a few hundred yards of warm-up make light dress just right. We're in the Rocky Mountains. The path winds out from the trailhead through a short stretch of flat ground, a gentle warm-up, and then the climb begins, a short uphill that catches you pushing a bit too hard and then your clean, aerobic heart rate spikes past the red line. You hold your pace for as long as you can, pitting will against slope, and then you're light-headed and winded and the quadriceps signal fatigue. Too soon for this. You're busted, and you walk. Heart rate recovers as you climb, head clears in a few hundred yards, and then you notice the hill has flattened at ridgetop to deliver a sweeping vantage of the valley below. You take it in, recover, and now trot. You measure your pace, tune it to the incline, and then again you are running. You don't let up but aim a steady climb for the first little summit you spot a hundred yards on. Now there's mud, and the trail becomes a trench, catching the melt of a winter's retreating snowdrift just above. More distress messages from quads and lungs, but you've got the pace right and hold it, light head be damned. And then you make that bit of a summit in a rush and a slight little giggle of triumph—first of the day—and then almost immediately sweep down the back side of the hill, shift gears, take it a bit too fast in skippy, quick steps, but it feels right, hopping rocks and roots, rocking off banked turns with a quick roll of the foot, vaulting puddles and little stubborn slicks of ice. The trail steepens and winds to a bend. You careen around the curve, bracing off rocks, and then spot a quick four-foot stair-step drop through a wall of rocks, step it, tick, tick, tick, splash in the mud below, then another bend and just beyond, the light signals the trail's bend into tree cover, where sun does not penetrate this early in the year. Now you're moving a bit too fast for control, and the next step places you on the high end of a foot-wide luge course of ice that ends in a bend above a rock-face cliff. Your feet look for grit and gravel of any kind, anything to slow your mad sliding scramble down. By all means do not panic now. Do not lock up and brake. Easy does it. Balance. Control. And just then your dog, who has been following you in all of this, decides, as she always does, that being behind you is not good enough, and she goes in for a quick pass on your cliff side by ducking between your feet, a canine foul of clipping. You get a half second to debate whether she goes over the cliff or you do, but then you notice you have bent one leg 90 degrees from the knee, just right, and the dog makes a quick move to expertly snake her way around your other leg, no foul. (Every animal knows way more than you do.) And you carry on, another grin, another little victory over the trail. And so on.

We've just given you a little slice of life, a description of maybe ten minutes of running on a mountain trail. In contrast, consider how we might describe ten minutes of running on a treadmill: Get on the treadmill, take a step, left foot, right foot. Repeat. Even the vicarious experience on the mountain trail, even reading along, invited more of your brain to come for the ride. With luck, our description of the mountain run engaged some of your mirror neurons, your sense of empathy. Even in the telling, it is information-rich and, as a result, engaging. So it is with the real thing.

This is not to say we are writing a prescription for mountain running as the single true and only heaven. Nonetheless, mountain running provides a great path to understanding an important element of productive exercise, and it may, in fact, be time to do away with the idea of an exercise routine. The term "exercise" is an artifact of our industrialized, regimented, domesticated lives. If the brain is to take full advantage of what we now understand about the importance of movement, then you don't have to exercise; you've got to move. You've got to be nimble.

SMARTER MOVES

The argument that humans were born to run in many ways makes running the ideal subject to serve as a doorway into a better understanding of motion and brain development in general. Running lies at the core of the human experience, but that deep connection has also, in recent years, produced a flurry of investigation and research across disciplines that give this topic a better platform than most for launching the broader discussion of the importance of movement. This is especially true because the general line of thinking got a huge leg up into the popular discussion with the work of Christopher McDougall and his groundbreaking book, *Born to Run*, which encourages barefoot running on evolutionary grounds.

Ask any physical therapist who practices in a running town, and you'll hear about McDougall's influence. Such clinicians are fond of claiming a real affinity for his work, simply because barefoot running has delivered so many injuries and thus ensured a steady flow of income. Barefoot running is their business model.

Press them further, though, as we have, and you will find out this is not so much a critique of McDougall's work or the idea behind it. The injuries accrue from a narrow reading of that research, particularly the assumption that barefoot running is all about, well, bare feet. It's not. But more tellingly, some physical therapists report that the injuries are accruing disproportionately to road runners, people who adopt minimalist shoes and then run serious mileage on consistent, flat, even terrain, the same surface and motion, step after step. Further, many people make the change too quickly and do not give their feet time to overcome a lifetime of bad form. The resulting injuries, then, are not a contradiction of the whole idea; they are a confirmation.

The rationale behind minimalist or barefoot running is this: humans evolved without shoes but also evolved running. A lot of it, on the order of a 10K every day. This dictated a body and movement built around what is called a midfoot or forefoot strike. The foot does not reach out ahead of one's body to land on its heel but, rather, tucks in under the body in a shorter, gentler stride. The long, heel-striking stride prevalent in competitive running became possible only with the introduction of heavily cushioned shoes. More important, that change in stride and shoes, while protecting the heel, shifted forces through ankles, knees, and hips, places not meant to take those forces, and as a consequence, runners become more, not less, injured in the long term — injuries that result from the shift in form allowed by artificially padded shoes.

This is an important principle that goes straight to the core and founding idea of this book: that shortsighted, simplistic, single-factor fixes — especially those that ignore the evolutionary design of our bodies — often create more problems than they solve. To some, this was the end of the story. Shoe companies, even the very ones that developed the heavily padded clunkers of the late twentieth century, got into the business of offering minimalist shoes: lightly padded, low-to-the-ground, slinky, lightweight bedroom slippers. Our culture, being what it is, thought this was the answer, that you fix a problem by buying a single product, be it shoe or pill, and people did buy them and made minimalist running shoes the fastest-growing category in the industry. And then many of these runners did nothing to change their running stride, but went straight out and started pounding pavement and treadmills and then lined up for physical therapists to fix a new set of problems. This is a cautionary tale for all of us, not just runners. A deeper reading of this idea is in order, and therein we might find some exquisite and marvelous detail to guide us through subjects beyond running.

Take, for instance, proprioception, to begin simply. It's a concept well within anyone's grasp, quite literally, and it's a good way to begin. Imagine yourself forced to navigate a dark room crowded with the usual obstacles, like furniture, tight turns, and a light switch across the room. First, you reach out and use proprioception to know where your hand is without seeing it, but you also use your sense of touch to gather information that feeds your brain, taps memories, and reconstructs a map of the room in order to steer your body toward the switch. Part of what is going on here is proprioception, the brain's ability to use signals from your hand to tell you where you are in space and where you should go. Proprioception is your brain's ability to know where your body parts are relative to one another at any given moment.

Also at work are the extraordinary abilities of the hands to gather information, the sense of touch and perception through touch that we rely on in activities like writing with a pencil, manipulating tools, playing the guitar, and foreplay. All of this feeds the brain in a sort of map, and not just of the hand. The surface of the brain contains almost literally a map of various points on our body, a diagram that the brain uses to build the sense of where we are in space. This map even speaks to priorities: our hands, our most important instruments for command of the sensory world, map out on the brain right next to our genitals, areas of maximum sensitivity staked out by evolution for good reason, and so the example of foreplay above is not nearly as frivolous as it might have seemed at first. Likewise, our feet are mapped next to our hands, signaling their importance in guiding us through space, in coordinating with the brain to maintain our sense of order, direction, and balance. The extraordinary sensitivity of our hands to guide us through a dark room ought to be equaled by the ability of our feet to guide us through the world—but, as with many of our evolutionary endowments, civilization has short-circuited the relationship, in this case with shoes. While it may not have been the intent, all that foam and gadgetry and those stiff soles robbed the feet of proprioception, and robbed our brains, our neural circuitry, of the refined information and information processing that directed us for millions of years.

With aging, we worry about matters such as cancer and heart disease or maybe even Alzheimer's taking us out or leaving us debilitated in a nursing home, but gerontologists say that a far more prosaic problem is a bigger one. The simple act of falling often breaks hips and legs and robs people of independence and mobility prematurely. We fall because we have lost our sense of balance, literally lost our way in the world, or, more to the point,

118 • GO WILD

have given it up by allowing the neural circuitry that oriented us to atrophy.

This is not to argue that we will solve all our problems simply by getting rid of shoes, or by wearing minimalist shoes. Rather, we offer this as simply one more case study in unintentional damage done by insulating ourselves from the real world. But this is just the beginning. We didn't tell you this, but we had you in minimalist shoes along that mountain trail, so at every twist and turn, your feet were playing a symphony of muscles and nerves to roll off rocks, bank off curves, accelerate, and brake. But this was about far more than feet. Each time you shifted gears from uphill to down or from straight to curve or to hop a rock, a new set of muscles came into play, or the same set of muscles shifted from push to pull, from expand to contract. Quads, calves, and hamstrings, sure enough, but also hips if your stride was right and the full girdle of muscles that wrap your abdomen—all engaged in not just the running but the breathing, the twisting and turning. And you didn't just run. On the uphills you pushed your heart well beyond its aerobic rate, held this as long as you could, then you walked, and suddenly a whole new set of muscles came on line.

Simply by engaging the real, rocky, rolling world and its variety of stresses and varied challenges, you have engaged the full range of muscular and neurological activity that evolved in places just like this. And more than muscles and neurons. Take, for instance, that little giggle you had after that long uphill slog, the summit experience, that little triumph over adversity and challenge. What lay behind that rush of elation was a squirt of biochemistry stimulated by the muscle activity but crucial to your sense of well-being and your brain. Doubtless dopamine was a part of this little reward, the rush that we try to replace with drugs and stimulants or try to re-create with prescription antidepressants. Here it is free for the taking. But here we can see the evolutionary logic behind it: these little rewards are evolution's way of keeping us going, of making us survive. Evolution has made provisions for our happiness, but to take advantage of them you've got to move.

DISCOVERING A NEW WAY TO MOVE

Matt O'Toole has always made his living on health and fitness, enjoying a twenty-five-year career that has, when we talked to him, taken him to the head of the international sports gear manufacturer Reebok. He is buff and tough, as you might expect, and he dresses in the athletic casual code common in the Reebok offices just outside Boston. Like Reebok itself, O'Toole has recently undergone something of a personal transformation.

"I had started a streak about nine years before [my transformation]. I was running every day and I decided to make that my form of exercise, because I was always finding that when I had a different routine I could easily break it. I would miss two or three days because of traveling. So I started this thing where I ran every day, so if I got a streak going, I would not break it. But what happened at the end of nine years, my body was actually a wreck. I had all kinds of back problems, knee problems. My back problem got so severe that my doctor told me I couldn't run anymore." It was an odd admission for a guy in the business of selling running shoes.

Running was probably not O'Toole's problem as much as was

the fact that he did it every day and did it in that flat, monotonous pattern of a street runner, a treadmill runner—but that's not our point here. The point is where O'Toole and Reebok went. He joined CrossFit, a worldwide formalized form of exercise that stresses a variety of movements: weight training, jumping, running, throwing, push-ups, pull-ups—all designed to involve the entire body, recruit all muscles, just as it recruits heart, lungs, and mind. Further, it is done in groups of people and is competitive, but not in the sense of team against team. Rather, there is a group ethic. You compete against yourself first and the group cheers you along, marks progress, forms a sort of community. We'll have lots more to say about the element of community in a later chapter, but for the moment, let's be reductionist and stick with the physical.

O'Toole's back problems simply went away with CrossFit. His new routine was so transforming that it has transformed Reebok itself. The corporation has consciously and explicitly moved away from the model that tied sales and promotion to professional athletic superstars in football, soccer, hockey, and basketball (sports in which most participation involves a couch and a flat-screen television). Instead, Reebok has specifically endorsed CrossFit and is basing its corporate direction on getting people off couches and into gyms.

But there needs to be a bit of disclosure here, especially because one of the authors' direct involvement with Reebok is part of this story. John is a paid consultant to Reebok, hired to help shape this transition and to guide a comprehensive program of exercise based in schools. O'Toole says that reading John's book *Spark* was every bit as important as CrossFit in shaping a new direction for Reebok.

Again, we're not offering CrossFit here as a prescription so much as it is an illustration. We hope you hear in our brief description of CrossFit an echo of our earlier conversation with David Carrier, the University of Utah biologist who has spent a career looking at topics like persistence hunting and movement. Remember, Carrier's ultimate point was that the human body is unique among the bodies of our close relatives, our fellow mammals, in not having a sweet spot, in having muscles and a supporting skeletal system designed for a whole variety of movements. We are, as we've said, the Swiss Army knives of movement, and CrossFit is one exercise program consciously designed to reflect that fact. There are others, specifically some forms of martial arts and even dance that are evolving to grasp this awareness of the human body. Our prescription does not necessarily lock you into a gym. It certainly doesn't lock you on a treadmill in front of a flat-screen.

In our conversation with O'Toole, another echo emerged in his description. Repeatedly, he cited the variety of activities as being among CrossFit's greatest attraction. This word "variety," if you recall, was also pivotal in our earlier discussions of food and nutrition, pivotal in our consideration of human evolution. A standout feature of humanity in evolutionary terms was the ability to adapt and thrive in a variety of environments facing a wide variety of challenges. Evolution tells us that this overarching condition of our deep ancestral past is also the foundation of our present well-being and happiness.

And, in fact, this idea can steer us toward a metric of sorts. Yes, we have shied away from a specific prescription in our arguments, preferring to lay out some general ideas like variety to guide you toward a personal program. We are not saying you must go to a gym and do so many reps of these and a half hour of those at this heart rate at that frequency wearing this brand of shoe and fueling on this sports drink and supplement. All well and good, but how do you know you're on the right track? Weight loss? Tighter abs and butt? Posture? IQ test? None of these. We've got a better one, and, in fact, O'Toole brought it up on his own, unprompted, during our conversation.

"With CrossFit I realized right away the reason I wanted to keep coming back was it was a lot of fun to be around these people and do things that I hadn't been doing and really challenge myself," he said. "The experience became a lot more positive, where with running it was, check the box, I have to do it. CrossFit was, hey, I might actually want to do this."

That's it. That you actually begin to look forward to that point in the day when you get to cut loose and move, that you want to do this. That's when you know you are on the right track, and don't give up until you are. We're telling you that whatever form of movement you do to stay healthy is not right until it gets to be fun. Enjoyable. Nor is this as squishy and nebulous as it might seem. Remember the pathways of biochemistry between muscles and brain. Much of that chemistry is wound up in building a better brain, but much of it is also wound up in rewards, in feeling better, in being attuned to your body's signals that tell you that you are okay, on the right path, and moving forward.

And then one thing leads to another; for O'Toole, it leads to a mountaintop. Although he described himself as "not an outdoor person," he nonetheless decided to mark his fiftieth birthday and the changes in his life by climbing Africa's Mount Kilimanjaro.

DEEPER LAYERS

Our description of the mountain run was, we argued, information-rich, but now is where we admit to rigging the argument a bit more than you may have noticed. As we said, the information contained in the actual run was at least several orders of magnitude greater than would fit on a page, a flood of data to the runner's brain. Nonetheless, there were a couple of simple facts embedded in our description that freighted far more meaning than you probably realized. Remember the dog? Remember how the dog almost knocked you off a cliff at a critical juncture and that this apparent conflict resolved itself by a quick movement instinctive to both dog and runner? In this nanosecond, the runner's brain was presented with a whole set of information way outside the box of the usual exercise routine; at bottom, there was a calculation and evaluation of the well-being of something outside himself, an animal he cared about and even loved. He first faced a moment of peril and then shared that peril with another being in a burst of empathy. Do I kick the dog off the edge of this cliff, or do I go off myself? Then a decision, and then survival. How important was this moment in enriching the experience? This question deserves examination in detail, and we will do just that in a subsequent chapter about empathy and caring and our brains. But first, we need to point out a few more elements of this run that foreshadow larger considerations. It was a mountain run, an experience in the real world. It included ice, rock, mountains, wind, sun, and sweeping vistas of grassy slopes and valleys. It was grounded in nature, which is our ancestral home, the context of human evolution. How much of the value the runner gained from this experience derived from that context? This question deserves its own chapter and will get one.

But this context raises another idea, and we will turn to this idea next. Nature is a valuable setting for our challenges because it just doesn't care about us and is all-powerful. The day that we described was relatively benign. There was sun and blue sky to soften the edges of ice and rock, but every mountain runner and trail runner knows that it could just as easily have been otherwise (and often is), that winds at ridges can summon blasts strong enough to knock you off your feet, or a weather front can blow in whiteout blizzards and temperatures plunging to subzero in a matter of minutes. What do you do about your run on such days? Do you gear up in the latest wonder fabric and press on? Some days, sure you do. There is value in facing a challenge that is real and has real consequences.

But think about our ancestors who faced such conditions routinely and without benefit of wonder fabric. Sometimes the right thing to do is press on, and sometimes it's better to hunker down, to retreat downslope to the cave and the fire and a circle of family, friends, children, and dogs curled in the corner in tight, heat-holding balls. And then it is time to sleep. You've got to move, and then you've got to rest.

5

Bodies at Rest

Why Sleep Makes Us Better

The writer Elizabeth Marshall Thomas may have the most privileged window into the wild life. As a child in the early 1950s, she accompanied her eccentric, wealthy parents on an expedition into a then-unexplored and unroaded region of southwestern Africa, the Kalahari, in what was among the first contacts by civilized people with the hunter-gatherers she calls Ju/wasi, otherwise known as the !Kung or San. These are the guys in the photo we showed you in our introduction. She lived among them for long periods and in a 2006 book, *The Old Way*, recorded her memories in exquisite detail, some of it greatly illustrative of the case we make, some of it enigmatic, puzzling, and even contradictory, as any account of the human condition must be. But at the moment, we focus on this recollection because of what it tells of the subject we now turn to: sleep.

A further safety measure is that everyone sleeps lightly and not at the same time. In the Ju/wa camp at night, someone always seemed to be awake, getting warm by a

fire or having a sip of water from an ostrich eggshell.…
The arrangement was very informal, not like a soldier's
guard duty or a sailor's watch. It just seemed to happen,
part of the normal way of life.

Normal for them, maybe: they were guarding against lions. But
what has this to do with us? Ultimately, this account steers us to the
context of the wild life, and how the wild taught us how to sleep.

Probably the best place, though, to begin asking about sleep
is in the noontime basement cafeteria of Boston's Beth Israel
Deaconess Medical Center. Lions are not an obvious presence in
the lunchtime rumble and chatter of a research hospital cafeteria, crowded with mostly scrubs-clad medical stars and up-and-
coming stars, as harried, caffeinated, and sleep-deprived as the
rest of us. No one knows more about this than our host at this
lunch, Robert Stickgold, one of the world's leading researchers
on sleep, who works out of a lab based at Beth Israel. Mostly
people call him Bob, which fits his informality and directness.
He is the sort of scientist who knows the data, and knows what
the data can and can't tell us, and what it can't tell us is the
answer to the most fundamental question: Why do we sleep?

"We understood the biological functions of the sex drive,
hunger, and thirst two thousand years ago, and for sleep we
didn't know it a dozen years ago, so the first thing I would suggest
is, it is subtle," he says. Nonetheless: "If you don't sleep, you die.
The rat work is very clear, but after twenty years [of studying
this], we don't know why the rats die. Cause of death unknown."

That's not the same as saying we don't know what will go
wrong if we don't sleep, just that it's not at all clear what it is
about this state of apparent mental and physical retreat, this lit-

tle death each of us must go through each day that serves our well-being. And what can go wrong for the sleep-deprived — we'll bet most of us are — ought to be front and center in the broader conversation. Here's a snippet from our conversation.

Stickgold: If you don't get enough sleep, you are going to end up fat, sick, and stupid.
Ratey: Which is the way the world is going anyway.
Stickgold: And that may be why.

Fat: Stickgold says the Iraq War, which consumed multi-trillions of dollars across the decade of American involvement, really ran on Snickers bars. As wars go, Iraq was a standout for a variety of reasons, but mostly it was an air war and mostly it was fought at night when American technology granted complete command of the dark. As a result, a lot of sleep was lost, which has prompted a great deal of research, especially by the military. Now we understand that one of the consequences of sleep deprivation is craving the very dense carbohydrates and sugars that featured so prominently in our discussion of nutrition. Researchers have since duplicated the phenomenon with studies that deprived volunteers of sleep.

"Put college students on four hours of sleep a night, and then give them a glucose tolerance test, and they look prediabetic. Food consumption goes up." This is insulin resistance, provoked solely by lack of sleep. Obesity and sleep loss have long been associated, but the research has zeroed in on the reasons why. For instance, in a study published after our conversation with Stickgold, researchers based at the University of Colorado found that sleep deprivation did indeed show a marked increase in weight gain, even with no measurable decline in activity or in energy expenditure. Instead, the experience disrupted the body's signaling pathways associated with the insulin response, particularly a set of hormones that signal satiety: ghrelin, leptin, and peptide YY. As a result, people ate more—especially women, especially in the evening.

Sick: Sleep deprivation seems to wreak havoc with the immune system, and this is not especially difficult to prove. Again, volunteers are sleep-deprived for just a few days, and then researchers give them and a control group a hepatitis C vaccination. The sleep-deprived people produce fully 50 percent fewer antibodies in response to the vaccine, a measure that says their immune systems are about half as effective.

This is what Stickgold means by subtle, in that most of us would never notice a compromised immune system, and most of us would never associate that cold with a lack of sleep.

"Is that going to kill you? Maybe. If it does, you are never going to connect the dots," he says.

Stupid: Well, yes, and just that directly. Reams of research and a variety of related ideas demonstrate this conclusively: Sleep-deprived people generally perform more poorly on straightforward skills tests, such as the ability to recall a list of facts. Subjects allowed to nap between learning the facts and taking the recall test do better. And this area of inquiry is what has made sleep science something of a growth industry. As the Snickers bars suggested, the military paved the way, but the front of this effort now is centered in the dollars-and-cents world of business. Sleep is just good business.

For instance, companies like Google, Nike, Procter & Gamble, and Cisco Systems have begun allowing employees to take naps at work as a way to enhance both productivity and creativity. Business consulting firms have capitalized on the research to show that sleep is essential to success.

On a simple and important level, all of this is a matter of competence, of simple ability to recall facts and solve problems, and indeed the work began aimed at those sorts of skills. Stickgold, for instance, is known for running labs full of subjects playing the popular video game Tetris and demonstrating that various combinations of sleep made them better at it. This is enough to fly straight in the face of the popular archetype of our culture drawn from Silicon Valley, where, legend tells us, fortunes were made by amped-up engineers writing code around the clock, never leaving the office and never taking a break. It is a dangerous stereotype. Still, it persists, and Stickgold has a way of challenging it directly. Students he knows who still buy into this idea of the caffeinated overachiever often boast of their ability to function on four or five hours of sleep each night. He suggests to them that they account for their time and performance, and they quickly figure out that the reason they need to work twenty hours a day is they are doing everything twice. They have to, because sleep loss is making them work inefficiently.

John encounters this problem in schools, especially when he is working in Asia. Kids are extremely sleep-deprived from staying up all night playing video games. They come to school and perform poorly, then are sent to special study halls at night, lose more sleep, then play more video games, and the downward spiral continues.

In fact, the research suggests that sleep has far more effect on far more complex skills, that it almost serves as a sort of retreat for our brains, a time to shut out extraneous noise and the rush of new information and, instead, sort through information to make sense of it. Seen in this light, sleep is a time for forgetting, for putting away what is not relevant, for pruning and sorting to allow the remaining information to form patterns and assist your brain in recognizing those patterns. This helps explain the almost legendary anecdotes about creative bursts and elegant solutions to complex problems that emerged spontaneously after a good night's sleep, the sort of thing that wins someone a Nobel Prize.

In our conversation, though, Stickgold raised a more mundane example of a common decision someone must make when offered a new and better job in a new town.

"The anal-compulsive person draws a chart: stay, go, pluses and minuses. It never helps. But then they wake up the next morning and say they can't take the job. And when friends say 'Why?,' they say, 'It's just not right for me,' and they can't tell you why."

The chart doesn't help because it can't include all the costs and benefits to the person and the spouse and the children and the weight of severed relationships and distance from family and the upheaval of disrupting a life. Not all of these can be neatly categorized and quantified, and even to the degree that they can, the calculation load becomes literally mind-boggling. The important judgments we make in our lives do not yield to lists of pluses and minuses and calculations. We settle these issues during sleep because that is when the brain seems best able to tackle the incalculable problems by pruning, consolidating, and synthesizing.

"One of Bob's aphorisms," says Stickgold, "is that for every two hours your brain spends taking in information during the day, it needs an hour of sleep to figure out what it means. If you don't get that hour, you don't figure it out. The difference between smart and wise is two hours more sleep a night."

This idea takes on a new dimension in the results of further research that appears at first to be a simple test of recall. Researchers showed subjects lists of images and then tested both people who were sleep-deprived and those who weren't on recall of the images. But these were images with clear emotional content, like a soft little puppy or an image of war, images sortable as negative, positive, or neutral emotionally. Of course, as we've already discussed, sleep-deprived people had some difficulty with recall, true enough, but not with the negative images. Those they could remember.

This finding is a slam-dunk link to depression. Almost by definition, depressed people are those who can remember only the negative aspects of their lives. The link goes further. For instance, people who suffer from sleep apnea, a common breathing malfunction that causes them to lose sleep, often also suffer from depression. But Stickgold says that one study, in which the apnea was successfully medicated and the depression was not, revealed that the depression corrected itself—showing that ensuring a good night's sleep cured the depression.

This phenomenon is especially pronounced in a particular area of emotional memory processing in those who suffer from post-traumatic stress disorder, a problem much larger than a Snickers bar habit for Iraq War veterans. One line of research demonstrated that people who were truck drivers during the war did not suffer nearly the levels of PTSD that other veterans did. This was because the military had a rule that truck drivers had to sleep eight hours in every twenty-four, and the rule was enforced.

We know now that PTSD is a creature of memory, a disease of memory. Sufferers are unable to process and assign their traumatic events to the past and so are condemned to relive these terrifying scenes day after day as real and present threats. Sleep's power over memory, however, can allow soldiers who have been through frightening and wrenching experiences to relegate them to their proper place in memory, where the events become just bad memories, not present threats.

So what do we do about all of this? Stickgold has a prescription and is, in fact, rather blunt about it: everyone needs eight and a half hours of sleep out of every twenty-four. Everybody. Further, it is more or less impossible to oversleep. That is, if you need an alarm clock to wake up every day, if you can't get rolling until after the third or fourth shot of espresso, and you find that you sleep long and hard on weekends, then you are probably not getting enough sleep. In this regard, the body is wonderfully homeostatic; that is, it has strong measures and mechanisms to enforce its need for sleep. It's almost as simple as this: if you are sleepy, sleep.

BEVERLY TATUM'S STORY

We met Beverly Daniel Tatum at Rancho La Puerta, a wellness retreat near San Diego that centers its methods on getting people back in touch with their better nature by putting them in contact with nature. But the path that brought her there began with a good night's sleep, and ultimately that path leads to the well-being of thousands of young women, because she is president of Spelman College. Tatum was taking one of her regular fitness breaks at Rancho La Puerta, part of her program to take care of herself so she can better do her job and take care of others, which she learned to do through direct experience.

Before she came to Spelman, Tatum was a dean at Mount Holyoke College, and that job placed some heavy demands on her time that she met by spending, as many of us do, too many late-night hours in front of a computer answering email. The emails multiplied when she became president of Spelman, a four-year college historically for African American women that's located in Atlanta, Georgia. So did the requisite official breakfasts, lunches, and dinners, which she calls "state dinners." So she was getting four or five hours of sleep a night, cutting back on her exercise, and she put on what she calls the "presidential twenty," not just the freshman fifteen familiar to many college students.

Tatum took a vacation in 2005 and realized that her weight gain was somehow tied to the long hours, just as Stickgold says—and she decided that she needed to take control. She set for herself a hard, fast rule to shut off her computer at 10 p.m. and go to bed. She slept at least seven to eight hours per night, regained her exercise habits, and soon began to lose some weight. She had more energy, felt better still, and saw that a lot of her students had the same problem she had had.

"I told them we're investing a lot in your education here," she said. "We want you to live long enough to get a return on our investment." Her dire warning was not conjecture. She had already learned that the obesity problem left her student body with high rates of diabetes and heart disease, to the point where she was going to the funerals of alumnae in their thirties.

So Tatum went ahead with a controversial decision to end Spelman's participation in the NCAA and organized collegiate sports, a move that made national news. Instead, she launched a comprehensive program of fitness and nutrition awareness campus-wide, designed to get students moving and eating well. And so twenty-one hundred students, future leaders, get the message and a better life, and this is how it builds. This is how change happens.

That path for change for Tatum began with a single step, which she calls a "lever." She pulled a single lever, and in her case, it happened to be sleep—but that gave her the foundation to embrace better nutrition and exercise. It all hangs together. And ultimately, her improved well-being manifested itself as service to the well-being of others. This is our model, and its context is nature, the wild.

THE SOCIAL CONTEXT

So sleep is good, but sleep how? In what environment? It turns out that the question of how is as relevant as how much. Much of the research has illuminated the complexity of sleep. We sleep in discrete stages, each marked by clear and distinctive patterns of brain activity. Further, some of these stages correlate with specific benefits. This means that a particular stage is necessary for learning or for memory consolidation, for instance, and if you disrupt sleep in ways that deprive a person of that specific stage, the benefits linked to that stage do not accrue, even if the total sleep is at the golden average of eight and a half hours per night. This shows that there is a quality issue at work here, and this is where we are left in the dark. We really don't know what normal sleep is, but we have some strong signals that the way we do it, a single, solitary, silent stretch, eleven until seven thirty, entombed in retreat from all others, is downright freakish behavior in terms of the human condition and human evolution. Might this habit of ours cause troubles? Maybe our dreams can tell us something about this.

At least when considered in one aspect, sleep is not a peaceful proposition. We dream about bad things. And the research on this matter is interesting: acts of aggression and threats and violence are overrepresented on our list of dream topics. We are more likely to dream about a thug threatening us with violence than a sunny day in a meadow with bunnies and butterflies. For instance, one study found that acts of aggression constituted about 45 percent of the dream content of one sample of people — by far the dominant dream category. In those cases, the dreamer was directly involved in the aggression about 80 percent of the time and was more often than not the victim. However, this burden of fright is not equally shared among all humans, although there are some common elements between genders and among adults. With both genders, the attacker in a violent dream tends to be a male or group of males or an animal, with animals in the minority, at least among modern adults.

This analysis gets far more interesting in the case of children, for whom the scary element tends to be overrepresented as animals. Further, the animal content of younger people's dreams tends to be skewed to the violent and threatening. Dogs, horses, and cats are underrepresented, while snakes, spiders, gorillas, lions, tigers, and bears make far more frequent appearances. More telling still, there is an age gradation to both of these factors. That is, dreams of situations involving threats from animals are more common among the very youngest children and taper gradually as children move toward adulthood. In effect, children—and this is true across cultures—slowly adjust their dream content to the realities of their world. It seems as if they are born afraid of attacks from aggressive animals and gradually substitute bad guys with sticks and guns for lions. But still, threatening situations are overrepresented.

That this is true, even of children who have never seen a wild animal and have no reason to fear an attack, suggests something quite innate, a hardwired memory of conditions more realistic in evolutionary time, when children and adults both had every reason to fear animal attacks. This can seem a bit preposterous to the modern, rational mind, but probably only because we are talking about dreams. There is plenty of nonsense, superstition, and speculation involved in the topic of dreams through the years, and so there's every reason to be suspicious. Nonetheless, there is a parallel and well-established phenomenon among the waking, and not just among humans but among other primates as well. Take a city-bred, born-and-raised denizen of concrete for his first walk through the desert, and then surreptitiously toss a live snake in his path. The reaction will be quick and predictable, regardless of whether your subject has ever seen a snake before. Same is true of chimps raised in cages. We have instincts, animal instincts, and this is demonstrable.

Yet even more interesting is the maintenance and sharpening of these very instincts among people living where the instincts come in handy, and this is borne out in the dreaming research as well. The closest we can possibly come to knowing about how our ancestors dreamed is through studies of contemporary hunters and gatherers, and it turns out that this has been done at least twice: once with aboriginals in Australia and once with the Mehinaku Indians of central Brazil, before there had been significant contact with the outside world. The latter case proved especially informative because these people actually valued dreams, so they were careful to note content and often talked about dreams with one another. In both Brazil and Australia, animals and aggression were overrepresented in dream content. In both countries, people dreamed about animals far more often than similar samples of civilized humans did, but at about the same rate as civilized children did, indicating that the decline of animals in dreams as we age is indeed an adjustment to our civilized, tamed world. We enter the world programmed to dream of the wild, but civilization takes those dreams away.

But just as important, the gender differences are alike among both hunter-gatherers and the civilized. In both cases, aggression and animals loom larger in the dreams of men.

Antti Revonsuo, who compiled and analyzed this large body of research in an important paper, concludes that this is really about something other than fear and trauma. Rather, it is far more in line with the main body of research on sleep in general. In his view, sleep is not a retreat to helplessness, but rather a functioning part of our learning process when the brain works through problems and devises solutions. Humans evolved among predators. Our formative years were not spent at the top of the food chain, a factor we think is too often glossed over in formulating the just-so stories about human evolution. Modern humans have forgotten what it is like to be meat, and being prey must have entailed terrors beyond imagination, particularly for the young and helpless and for the people who cared about them most.

We can begin to imagine this state of being through extrapolation, especially those of us who have seen lions or grizzly bears or Siberian tigers in the wild (all, in fact, still posing a significant threat to some humans). And yet these animals were far more numerous during humanity's history than they are now, and they were joined or preceded by even more formidable predators, now extinct. For instance, modern-day !Kung people fall prey more often to leopards than to lions, but ancestor leopards of that place were in fact much larger, giant leopards, with every bit the speed and prowess of the more compact variety that still kills people. Even North American native people encountered saber-toothed tigers and short-faced bears, which were larger and faster than modern grizzly bears.

In such an environment, skills for dealing with predators would have been highly adaptive, to say the least, and that is exactly what determined the content of our dreams. Revonsuo believes that dreams served as a rehearsal of challenging events, to allow our brains to work at night on the reactions and skills necessary to deal with our most important threats. He concludes:

> Any behavioral advantage in dealing with highly dangerous events would have increased the probability of reproductive success. A dream-production mechanism that tends to select threatening waking events and simulate them over and over again in various combinations would have been valuable for the development and maintenance of threat-avoidance skills. Empirical evidence from normative dream content, children's dreams, recurrent dreams, nightmares, post-traumatic dreams, and the dreams of hunter-gatherers indicates that our dream-production mechanisms are in fact specialized in the simulation of threatening events, and thus provides support to the threat simulation hypothesis of the function of dreaming.

Carol Worthman, meanwhile, believes that the presence of predators also formed our habits of sleeping, which steers us in another direction, toward the flip side of fear. If we look closely, we can find ample evidence that sleep is not retreat but an act of social engagement, and this, too, can be derived from wondering where the lions are.

Worthman is an anthropologist and probably the only one in captivity who specializes in sleep. We caught up with her at Emory University; she's a polite and engaging woman in a neat and fully organized office. She had just returned from a stint in India teaching the scientific method to Buddhist nuns and a stop in Vietnam to check on research in a remote village where television had been introduced for the first time.

Years ago, Worthman tackled the topic of sleep, mostly out of curiosity and her wonder as to why there was not more on the subject in the anthropological literature, given the importance of sleep in our lives. She did a survey of cross-cultural research on sleep habits and found, much as Stickgold found in research on the reasons for sleep, that we know almost nothing. There is some excuse for this. People sleep in private, or at least we once assumed so. Further, unlike spear tips and hand axes in hunting and fire smudges in cooking, sleep leaves no trace in the archaeological record, not much in stories, and not much in our bones — and so there is precious little to go on if we need to ask the very question about sleep that we have been asking in this book about other endeavors, like food and movement: what is the evolutionary history of this fundamental human activity?

It turns out that the anthropological perspective does nothing to contradict Stickgold's conclusions from studies of modern-day sleepers, but it does provide a different emphasis, especially on the prescription. There is nothing in the cross-cultural studies that disagrees with the idea of the need for a baseline of sleep of about eight hours out of every twenty-four, but Worthman says her real concern is with quality, not quantity. For instance, she says people who complain about insomnia—the torturous variety that has one lying in bed awake, tossing and turning through the night—often sleep far more than they report, but they get only low-quality sleep. They believe they are awake—and, more to the point, the sleep they do get doesn't do them a lot of good.

"The question is how do you get good sleep, and that draws attention to context, and that's where the evolutionary context can be helpful," Worthman says.

What we know about evolutionary context is extrapolation from what we know from cross-cultural sleeping habits. But nonetheless, the studies contain some clear evidence that we are missing something important about context, at least we who practice what Worthman calls the "lie down and die" model of sleep: to bed at ten, lights out, silence, set the alarm, and await resurrection. The simple fact is, across the world and across time as far as we know, few cultures sleep this way.

"In virtually all societies there is a sense of the social organization of sleep, and in many, many societies the provision of an appropriate sleep context is viewed as extremely powerful," she says.

And what does an appropriate context look like? To begin with, it includes other people. Few other cultures view sleep as a retreat, even a private act. Just the opposite.

Back to the lions for a moment, to see where that comes from. Thomas described a scene as much about being awake as it was about being asleep, which makes perfect sense if you happen to be a !Kung sleeping outside among lions, and through most of evolutionary time, humans did indeed sleep outdoors among predators. But there is actually some math at the root of this casual observation, calculations that Worthman has done. This is based on well-known and established variations in sleep patterns that remain fixed in modern humans, according to age. Babies can be and often are awake at seemingly random periods around the clock, but once they are a bit older, they lock onto a circadian rhythm much like that of adults. Adolescents, however, have a rhythm of their own, worldwide and across cultures: they go to bed late and get up late, compared with adults. Older people, meanwhile, are often awake longer and for periods in the night. This age segregation is consistent across cultures but begins to make sense when one superimposes those various patterns on one another. Worthman says that doing so allows a calculation that, given a band size of about thirty-five people with usual age distributions, yields a group pattern in which at least one person is awake at any given time.

Yet there is more to this than simply being awake. Many cultures, for instance, cultivate a form of light sleep, a watchful doze that is instantly reversible. In the studies of modern sleepers, this corresponds with a stage of sleep that confers a distinct set of benefits. Everyone performs this sort of light sleep without realizing it, but each of us also needs periods of very deep sleep, a stage vital to brain benefits and at the same time deeply threatening to people who live among lions. Researchers generally divide sleep into two categories by eye movement: rapid eye movement, or REM, sleep and non-REM sleep. The latter category has four distinct stages. Both REM sleep and the deepest stage of non-REM sleep are marked by a near complete lack of muscle tone and awareness; it's like being in a coma, helpless against threats like predators.

In REM sleep, debilitation is nearly complete. Two pathways of brain chemistry work together to induce paralysis in all muscles but the eyes. Researchers don't know the function of this paralysis but speculate that it prevents injury caused by muscles acting out our dreams, which also mostly occur in the REM state. People with disorders that prevent this paralysis often suffer such injuries.

Worthman says these stages, more than even the threat of lions, are why the social context of sleep is vitally important. We are not checked out or mentally absent during sleep, at least not all the time. On the contrary, as the research has shown, our brains are doing some of their heaviest lifting during sleep. But doing that requires modulation, a shifting of gears from one stage of sleep to another, which in turn requires some attention to context, reading of the signals that tell us when it is safe to check out and become helpless against external threats. In order to sleep properly, we need to pay attention to what is going on around us, using that awareness to guide us through the necessary stages of sleep. Isolating ourselves in soundproof rooms may be about the worst way there is to go about this—but, more to the point, so is isolating ourselves from other people.

This conclusion is not speculation. Worthman carried out one research project in Egypt, which gave her access to subjects who have been settled in cities for millennia. The choice was deliberate: she wanted to look at the persistence of hunter-gatherer sleep patterns, despite civilization. Egyptians, in both city and countryside, sleep the way most of the world does, which is to say together—what she calls "consolidated sleeping." Typically, whole extended families sleep in great rooms, with almost no isolation. There are exceptions, though, and those proved to be the most telling. Egyptians and others typically segregate post-pubescent girls from boys. Not always. Sometimes there is an aunt or grandmother and the teenage girl bunks with her. But some end up sleeping alone, and it was those people, both boys and girls, who had the insomnia and other forms of dysregula-tion. The people who slept alone had the emotional problems.

This same pattern has emerged in a variety of studies to the point that we begin to understand why social sleeping seems to be a nearly universal characteristic of cultures, as are the stag-gered patterns of wakefulness of the group. While we are sleep-ing, we continue to monitor our surroundings for cues of safety: relaxed conversation, relaxed movement of others, popping fire. Those cues, subtle sounds signaling safety, tell us we can retreat to our deepest sleep.

Many cultures are, in fact, conscious of all of this and the importance of these arrangements, and no place is the impor-tance more pronounced than in the case of infants. (We need not necessarily bring lions into the picture to underscore this, although predators like hyenas and leopards are certainly prefer-ential to the young of our species, undoubtedly one of the rea-sons infant mortality was high among our ancestors. Thomas, for instance, records one example of great injury to a toddler who stumbled into a campfire while others were sleeping, and this was probably a common occurrence through time.) One of the biggest reasons for modulated sleep is to protect infants.

But the research suggests that this works in both directions—that is, infants' bodies are instinctively aware of their vulnerabil-ity and so do things like dream about frightening animals. They are even more dependent than adults on signals of safety. All of this helps explain what Worthman characterizes as an almost universal perplexed response among most other cultures upon hearing of the Western practice of making babies sleep alone.

"They think of this as child abuse. They literally do," she says.

The evolutionary context of sleep, however, extends well beyond the people around us, and this may begin to suggest some antidotes to our present isolation, some practical steps one might take to reintroduce evolutionary context to our rest. Anthropological studies have shown that almost all cultures pay a great deal of attention to the sound of a fire, and not just as a threat to babies. Changes in the crackle and pop might, for instance, signal that a fire is dying and trigger a new level of alert sleeping, just as the sounds of a fire settling into a sustained glow might signal that it's okay to sleep deeply. This doesn't mean you need to sleep next to a fire (although it's nice if you can). But you can look for similar patterns of sound that may help, even recordings.

Likewise with animals. Herders in particular sleep with such sounds as cud chewing and gentle bovine breathing, signals from sentinel animals of peace that transpires when no predators are around. Our favorite sentinels through evolutionary time were once predators: wolves slowly tamed by food to be dogs. Any suburban dweller can attest how the sound of an incessantly barking dog can be profoundly disturbing to sleep, more than decibels and persistence alone can account for. Yet we forget how the reverse is certainly true: that many of us tune our degree of peace and relaxation to the rhythms of a snoring dog. If something were wrong, the dog would say so.

All of this may be enough to explain the finding of epidemiology that people who are married and people who have pets live longer. It may be because they sleep better.

AGAIN, VARIABILITY

In one of her papers, Worthman wrote something that circles this whole idea back to fat, sick, and stupid. Like Stickgold, Worthman is deeply impressed with the homeostatic nature of sleep, that the body has an overwhelming sense of needing it and, left to its own devices, will do what must be done to ensure adequate sleep.

It's a wonderfully fluid phenomenon, she says, which is why most cultures don't worry about sleep or even losing sleep. If you're awake tending the fire or sheep one night, no big deal: doze through the afternoon and catch up.

She's seen conversations like a business negotiation among, say, a group of men in Egypt that conclude when one guy simply falls asleep.

"Literally, a guy will just pull a cloth over his head and go to sleep," she says. "And that's no biggie. It's not like a guy just slid under his chair in the boardroom. It's not asocial. If you view sleep as a social behavior, then it is just integrated in life."

But this is only true if our bodies are left to their own devices, and our rushing, wired world has all sorts of devious mechanisms for overriding those controls. That's the dilemma. How do we get away with this, this deficit that accrues not just for a couple of days but day in and day out, through whole careers? Where is homeostasis? How do our bodies balance this behavior?

Worthman's answer is this: we pay for sleep deficit in the currency of stress.

"Sleep deprivation looks like stress. It increases cortisol, it increases appetite, decreases satiety, increases blood glucose levels," she says. "This is straight out of the stress literature. If you curtail sleep just now and then, you can manage the hit, but if you do it too much, it erodes the health of the organism, the person, and her ability to cope."

This, too, is a case for modulation and adaption. On the one hand, sleep is far more elastic than we make it out to be. Indeed, it is wrong to characterize it as inactive or in retreat. Rather, it is a dynamic state important to brain function and some of our most important work. More to the point, sleep is when we *do* some of our most important work, both in processing information and, as the cultural studies show, in engaging others and building social bonds of trust. And because it is so important, it is adaptable and fluid. That is, our bodies are hardwired with a series of circuits to allow sleep to flow with the needs and demands of our day, what Worthman means when she calls it "fluid." And as with most other cases of our adaptability, we need to practice adapting to strengthen that skill, to modulate, to read the signals and cues that attach us to our physical and social environment, flexing the adaptive tools like muscles.

This is just like the response to stress that makes us stronger in exercise, that is unless that stress becomes chronic and unremitting, day in and day out, and then we pay in the currency of cortisol and inflammation: fat, sick, and stupid. Complete recovery of the evolutionary context of sleeping is probably lost to us, but we have the basics. We probably don't know enough and have lost the proper environments to make sleep perfect, but at least we have some clues as to how to make it better. That and ample evidence that we ought to do so.

For many of us, this is a simple matter of ensuring sufficient sleep, the fundamental issue in our overstimulated, overcaffeinated lives. It is true that much about sleep and sleep disorders remains a mystery, especially when we begin considering the evolutionary rules, as we have here. But one important fact we know for sure is that you must get sufficient sleep, and way too many of us don't.

Beyond this, evolution provides some hints about the proper context of sleep: Irregularity is okay. So are naps. A sense of safety is critical. If you can, sleep around others, and this may include traditional sentry animals like dogs. Some people have even found that the relaxed sounds of conversation typical of all-night radio do the trick. Avoid alarming sounds like sirens. Look for safe sounds like the lapping of gentle waves (a signal of safe weather, no storms) or a settling wood fire. Try recordings if you can't be near the real thing.

And then there is light, and in this there is an intriguing clue that suggests we have so much to learn. Much has been made of this issue of light as it affects our sleep, and the advent of artificial light is right up there with agriculture as one of the more profound shifts in the conditions of our existence, particularly for those humans who ventured north and south to where day's and night's lengths vary widely.

Of course, we can argue that artificial light has been with us a very long time; we've already talked about the importance of fire. The famous cave painters at places like Lascaux and Chauvet had fat-fueled lamps that they used to execute their artwork as long as forty thousand years ago. But fire and fat produce light of very different wavelengths than electric lights do and, more to the point, much dimmer light. This is key. The real problem is light bright enough to mimic the sun. Virtually all living organisms, even plants, are finely tuned to cycles of light and dark, to the passing of days, but also of seasons, patterns of life called circadian rhythms. Evolution has embedded layers on layers of mechanisms in humans to honor these cycles, and there has been plenty of research into at least one of these layers to tell us light is pivotal, not just to sleep but to our health and longevity in general.

The mechanism is pretty simple. Sunlight strikes a tiny gland behind the eye called the pineal gland, which in turn regulates the production of melatonin, the hormone that governs sleep and our circadian rhythms. Any artificial light that approaches the brightness of the sun is enough to trigger this same process, and the research shows that the everyday, garden-variety 100-watt lightbulb is enough. The average office is about three times as bright as the threshold. The effect ratchets up with certain wavelengths, especially those that produce blue light, which takes us to electronic devices and televisions, all of which mess with melatonin. The blue wavelengths are accented in these devices, as they are in any light-emitting diodes (LEDs), such as those in super-energy-efficient lightbulbs. Research has already demonstrated a clear effect of computer monitors on melatonin, largely because of the specific wavelengths emitted.

Yet the effect of even the simple lightbulb goes a lot farther. Electric light conquered the night and made things like shift work possible, allowing people to work around the clock. Even those not working are more active than our ancestors, creating cities that never sleep and a regimen of noise that is unavoidable and takes a toll on our rest. Thus it gets hard to sort out the root cause of the damage—noise or light—but also the answer to this question: is the damage caused by lack of sleep or by disruption of the powerful circadian rhythm?

Nonetheless, the damage is there, and the studies bear this out. Nurses who work night shifts, for instance, are more likely to develop breast cancer. That same group had a 35 percent greater chance of suffering colon cancer. Studies have linked the disruptive effects of artificial light at night to depression, cardiovascular diseases, diabetes, and obesity. We believe that light is an enormous factor in problems like attention deficit disorder. And while it may be difficult to control the social conditions of sleeping for some people in some situations, most of us have much more control over light. An effective intervention here might be as simple as dimming all the lights and shutting down the television and computer monitor a few hours before bedtime. Another might be as drastic as finding a different job if the current one makes you work at night. But when weighed against issues like an elevated risk of colon cancer, such measures seem less drastic.

It's important to stress here that we are not arguing against exposure to light that mimics the sun, which would be like arguing against the sun. The problem here is timing, not exposure. Thus, the goal is to control the timing of our exposure to light to mimic the natural cycle of day and night and of seasons. This prescription, then, links with ideas we will raise later about the benefits of exposure to nature. Spending time outdoors in sunlight is as important as turning off lights at night to harmonize your body's circadian rhythms with the earth. This helps not just with sleep but with the full range of your body's finely tuned systems.

But go back for a moment to the idea of the second sleep for yet another link to other matters. Interestingly enough, some experiments in removing subjects from the influences of all artificial light have been done, just to see what would happen. In a matter of days, a pattern emerged in many subjects. They could sleep when they wished, and many adopted a habit of going to sleep early, say at eight o'clock, then would awake around midnight or so for a few hours, and then would go back to sleep—a bifurcated pattern of sleep. But what was intriguing about this was a parallel pattern that appears in writings from preindustrial Europe, a pattern of this "second sleep." Historically, people would use that interim period as quiet, thoughtful time, or for having sex, or even for going to visit neighbors. It was social time and it appeared naturally on body clocks set by the absence of artificial light. Researchers have also found similar patterns in various cultures.

There are a couple of key lessons in this intriguing fact. First, it tells us that our bodies are strongly hardwired for a specific and important behavior, and if we remove the artificial meddling of industrialism like electric lights, our systems will self-correct. We think this principle applies to a lot more than just sleep.

But there is a second clue here. That interim period between first and second sleep has a biochemical signature: elevated levels of the hormone prolactin. Prolactin shares a common etymological root with lactation and lactose because it was first identified, along with oxytocin, as a dominant hormone of breastfeeding, of lactation in mammals. Oxytocin especially has since gotten a reputation as the social hormone, as we shall see in a later chapter.

But prolactin shows up prominently in another context, among people who practice meditation—the topic we engage next.

6

Aware

What Is Revealed in the Wild Mind

A couple of decades ago, the anthropologist Richard Nelson told us an anecdote that seemed to say a lot then—and even more now, knowing, as we do, so much more about the mind. Nelson is one of those maverick researchers who became an anthropologist not because he was attracted to academia but because he'd rather live in remote places among wild people. His particular chosen station early on was living among Koyukon people, caribou hunters of the frigid interior of Alaska. Later, though, he chose to live in the very different environment along the coast, the warmer maritime archipelago of islands that Alaskans call "Southeast." This is a place of rain, cedars, seals, and salmon, the interior a place of Arctic winters, fur, wolves, and ice.

Several of the Koyukon became Nelson's friends, and after he had lived some time in Southeast, he decided to invite a few of them to visit him at his new home. He expected a reunion—swapping stories, laughs, and endless rounds of warm conversation. But when they arrived on the island where he lived—a place wholly unfamiliar to them—they gave him only silence.

They were struck near dumb by the overwhelming detail in the strangeness all around them, and they wandered the island absorbing every sodden green inch of the place. After days of this, they could at last speak, and they proceeded to describe to Nelson his own island home in far more detail and with far more insight than he could after years of living there.

This is the hunter-gatherer state of mind, a hyperawareness, a presence, a capacity for observation we can only begin to imagine. The authors have some inkling of what it means and where it comes from as a result of deep personal experience. Richard Manning is a lifelong hunter, with almost fifty years' experience stalking game in the woods. Most of his household meat supply is hunted game. Even after a year at a desk, tethered to a computer and a cell phone, Richard finds that the hunting experience can summon forth a state of mind like no other. We had one watershed conversation about this, and oddly, although John has never hunted, the concept snapped into focus much of John's thinking about noise — mental noise — and mindfulness. Yet we think this modern experience of hunting is the merest approximation of the heightened powers of observation and awareness that were a fact of everyday life for the Koyukon and for all wild people. Generally, this mindful state is regarded as an ephemeral phenomenon that will not yield to hard-science, data-based analysis. Yet we think that mindfulness plays a large role in forming this common and wistful assessment by field researchers who have spent time among wild people: there is an otherworldliness and peacefulness to their lives we can but begin to imagine.

Through time, we have come to think there is a rough draft parallel to the hunter-gatherer mind-set that can be found in a modern-day practice—a practice that is in fact readily available to us and has been studied in detail, especially in recent years with the emerging tools of neuroscience. We are going to have a look at the formal practice of meditation as it emerged from Buddhist tradition. The thing is, the Koyukon hunters in our anecdote were not practicing meditators, as far as we know, and in this chapter, we are far more interested in the Koyukon state of mind than in meditation. We are, however, going to talk some here about formal meditation and the research behind it because we believe it illuminates the more general mind-set of hunter-gatherers. Later, we will link back to this general state of mind in ways applicable to modern people, meditators or not.

THE SCIENCE DEVELOPS

Richard Davidson began meditation quietly in the 1970s, when people training in serious disciplines like psychology at serious universities like Harvard didn't go in for this sort of idea. To complicate matters, serious psychologists also did not talk about emotion back then, and that's what happened to capture Davidson's interest.

"Overall, though, there just wasn't much room for emotions in the cold, hard calculus of cognitive psychology, which considered them downright suspect," Davidson wrote in his book *The Emotional Life of Your Brain*. "The attitude was basically one of haughty disdain that this riffraff occupied the same brain that gave rise to cognition."

Davidson latched onto an emerging tool then absent in psychology departments: the electroencephalogram, or EEG, which measures activity in various parts of the brain. He wanted to track the physical manifestations of emotion in the brain, but also other measures like heart rate and respiration. The concept was to link human behavior to a real, physical set of responses in the body. This was the line of thought that would lead to mapping the neural pathways of emotion.

During this period, Davidson was mostly mum about meditation in his professional life but was nonetheless pursuing the idea in some interesting social circles, arguably in the very house in Boston that served as a focal point for science's distrust of practices like meditation. Davidson's original contact at Harvard was the psychology professor David McClelland, who a decade earlier had run the research center that supported two faculty members, Richard Alpert and his coinvestigator, Timothy Leary, of LSD fame. When Davidson joined this circle in 1972, Alpert was by then known as Ram Dass and was living in the carriage house behind McClelland's house and teaching meditation. Davidson began a meditation practice then and followed that thread to India for formal training while he was still in graduate school.

Still, he kept that practice out of his work and instead chose to study emotions like fear, anxiety, and depression. He gained some new ground there, publishing some of the original work that tied those emotions to specific, identifiable parts of the brain, using tools like the EEG. But Davidson says that part of the reason he did not pursue research in meditation was because the tools of neuroscience were then not up to the task. And part of his reluctance was undoubtedly encapsulated in the phrase he uses for finally reversing that decision and beginning specific lab work on meditation. In his book, he labels this reversal "coming out of the closet."

It was indeed a dramatic exit from that closet, involving trunk loads of computer gear, electrodes, generators, and battery packs that had to be lugged by literal Sherpa guides on foot for days on end on treacherous, cliff-edge mountain passes; he was seeking out swamis, mystics, and gurus. No, really. Davidson launched an expedition near Dharamsala, India, attempting to find and wire the brains of some of the most experienced meditators on earth, those associated with Tibetan Buddhism. These were, Davidson allows, truly odd people, like Olympic athletes of the mind, in his analogy. They were far removed from the common experience, which is precisely why he sought them out. They are outliers, and it is interesting to consider how their extreme example might inform the rest of us.

Davidson, however, failed in this mission—but it led to nothing less than a challenge in 1992 from the current Dalai Lama, Tenzin Gyatso himself, who had become engaged in the process. Tenzin Gyatso challenged Davidson to bring to bear on meditation the same rigorous elucidation his EEGs had brought to his study of emotions.

Davidson was by then at the University of Wisconsin–Madison, where he remains, as a professor of psychiatry and psychology and the director of the Center for Investigating Healthy Minds at the Waisman Laboratory for Brain Imaging and Behavior. He used the challenge and the network of Tibetans he had come to know to eventually entice a handful of meditators, all of them experienced in the Tibetan Buddhist tradition, to his lab to have their brains wired. And they were indeed Olympic athletes of the practice. Each had logged at least ten thousand hours of meditation. Each had lived at least one three-year period in retreat, which means doing nothing but meditation every day, eight hours a day, for three years, never leaving the retreat site. One monk had spent more than fifty thousand hours in meditation. If meditation does indeed change the brain, then it ought to be obvious in these people. And it was.

By then, the more advanced brain imaging tools available through functional magnetic resonance imaging had come into play, so Davidson's lab could be a lot more specific about brain activation than he could have been with EEGs, which measure only surface activity of the brain. The researchers loaded the monks in fMRI tubes and had them meditate, not meditate, and meditate in various ways. They also played distressing sounds (like a woman screaming) for the monks at various unannounced intervals to record reactions. Researchers used similar routines for control subjects.

What they found was that the monks reacted much more to the screams than the control subjects did, and in a particular area of the brain—at the temporal parietal junction, which is strongly associated with empathy and the ability to take the perspective of another. This result occurred when monks were both meditating and not meditating. Davidson says the differences between the monks and the controls were not subtle, and the researchers had not expected such emphatic results, having long experienced the delicacy of brain waves and the difficulty of reading them. Normally, differences—even significant differences—are barely readable, or readable only with computer enhancement and amplification.

"We were absolutely stunned because the changes were so

robust and so dramatic that we were able to observe them with the naked eye, which is almost never the case in this kind of research," Davidson said in one interview about the work. "We can literally see the signal in front of us."

The problem was, the results really didn't answer the fundamental question: does meditation indeed change the brain? There's a perfectly good alternative explanation, which is that these people were somewhat freakish to begin with, given their long history of behavior that most of us would not even consider. Further, even if meditation can make a brain better and more empathetic, who has ten thousand hours to spend in a cliffside cave?

The monks' results only suggested a direction for research; the more interesting results have come in the twenty years since, as Davidson's lab has recruited and randomized samples of volunteers, taught them meditation in short courses, and loaded them in the fMRI tubes as well. Among the findings were clear and readable patterns in brain activation and reduction in anxiety and depression, but also some results you might not expect. During one experiment, researchers gave both meditators and control groups a flu vaccine and found a better immune response among the meditators, even the novices. Davidson's lab has subsequently shown a marked improvement among meditators who are undergoing a standard treatment for psoriasis, further establishing the brain-body connection. Specifically, meditators healed at about four times the rate that controls did.

"We did the study twice because we didn't believe the results," Davidson says.

Yet in all of this, there are some intriguing results that point toward the idea that brings us to this topic: meditation in some way mirrors the state of mind among hunter-gatherers. The common perception is that meditation is a state of retreat or withdrawal, much like the common perception about sleep that Carol Worthman's work contradicts. With meditation, the misinformed assumption is that the practice is aimed at relaxation and bliss. It is not. It is about attention and awareness of the here and now, which is precisely what wild people need in order to survive in a state of nature.

And, in fact, Davidson has done experiments that begin to illuminate this point. For instance, there is the matter of what is called the attentional blink. Each of us, no matter how we live, is perpetually immersed in a fast-moving stream of information, and it is up to us to pick out what is relevant from the stream to function, to recognize a threat or an opportunity or a clue that a game animal lies ahead or a child might fall or a potential client just walked in the door. Psychologists have a standard test for this: they read off a stream of letters and numbers in random order and ask people to respond whenever they hear a number but not a letter. It turns out that people are good at this simple task most of the time, but not when a number follows another number closely. The assumption is that the mental energy reserve they expend identifying the one target needs time to recharge, like a camera flash with rapid-fire photos. Those with weaker "batteries" miss the number that follows closely, causing an attentional blink.

In Davidson's experiments, meditators performed better, with less attentional blink, showing that this is not a matter of bliss or relaxation but of awareness and competence.

The improved perception is a benchmark of meditation; the benchmark is known from some of the earliest experiments, and the results are robust enough to become recognized as a neuro-logical signature of meditation. The meditative state is character-ized by synchronized gamma waves throughout the brain. "Gamma" simply means that they are of high frequency compared with other brain waves, but it is their synchrony that is more interesting. As you can imagine, the brain is driven by a cacopho-nous mix of waves and signals blasting away at all frequencies and in all directions, the exact picture presented by an EEG of an active mind. It looks like a sound wave pattern of street noise, and a chaotic street at that. But there is understandably a profound effect when those waves settle into a common, synchronous pat-tern, analogous to an orchestra's transition from the chaos of tun-ing to playing a root, third, and fifth of a chord in unison.

The term "neural pathways" makes us think of our brain as a sort of circuit board, where miniature wires connect one cell to another to make that path. An even more apt analogy for this profound effect is to imagine each neuron or cell as a radio that can be tuned to receive certain frequencies, to respond to a cer-tain wavelength generated somewhere else in the brain. Synchro-nous waves recruit bigger neural networks because more cells are tuned to that "station." Davidson calls it "phase-locking."

When a brain is wandering in noise, unsynchronized, "the response to an external stimulus is as difficult to pick out against this background cacophony as the ripples from a rock splashing into a turbulent sea. There are so many other waves and distur-bances that any ripples from the thrown rock are almost imper-ceptible. But if the rock lands in a perfectly still lake, the ripples stand out like a walrus in a desert. A calm brain is like a still lake," he writes in *The Emotional Life of Your Brain*.

This is not a matter for meditation alone but a concept

rooted in much thinking about mental well-being and mental illness. Think of it as noise, as we long have—not literal noise but analogous: meaningless rumble, chatter, and static in the backdrop of the brain like the conversation-killing roar of a busy restaurant. It is implicated in problems including schizophrenia, manic-depressive disorder, autism, mental retardation, and brain damage. People afflicted with these problems are often unable to control the rush of stimuli, to still the lake. What they suffer from is just the opposite. The noise arrives in a sort of mental echo chamber that ratchets up the racket to an unbearable level and provokes behaviors we call pathological. These behaviors are an attempt to cope with the noise. Some of John's early work on this idea found that calming the body in various ways served to calm this storm, a connection of physical to mental. But meditation also stands as a more direct attempt to calm the background of the mind—not to retreat, but as a way to allow the mind to more directly attend.

It is this state of awareness that brought us to the evolutionary roots of this matter in this discussion, but the question is, what has this to do with our present world? What is the importance of this awareness? We've already cited increased competence, and that is certainly enough to merit our attention, but there's a great deal more going on here.

LINKS TO STRESS

There was a remarkable gathering of minds in 2005, an interdisciplinary conference, and the conversation was recorded in a book edited by Jon Kabat-Zinn and Davidson called *The Mind's*

Own Physician: A Scientific Dialogue with the Dalai Lama on the Healing Power of Meditation. We recommend it as an interesting rundown of the confluence between neuroscience and mindfulness, summarizing what we know and speculating where we might go with this idea. It offers many remarkable insights— and not just into meditation but also into the more general and all-encompassing idea of mindfulness. For instance, at the conference, Helen Mayberg, a professor of psychiatry at Emory University, traced depression to detailed neural pathways, and she showed how those pathways changed through not meditation but cognitive behavior therapy—another way in which the mind reshapes the brain.

But the discussion was expanded significantly by the inclusion of Robert Sapolsky, the Stanford neurologist who has made a name for himself as the go-to guy on stress. The foundation of his work is tracking stress through the hormone cortisol, which has emerged as the accepted biomarker of stress. Sapolsky's most famous subjects were baboons living in the wild in Africa. He captured them periodically to measure cortisol in blood samples and discovered that the life of a wild animal could indeed be loaded with stress, the very factor we associate with the noise and rigors of civilized, human life. Sapolsky concluded that baboons suffered this same problem for much the same reason we do, and it had little to do with scarcity or predation. It actually arose from hierarchy. Baboon society is dominated by aggressive males who enforce dominance with violence and more or less constant harassment of subordinates. (Both leaders and subordinates wind up suffering from chronic stress, but in different ways.) One need not get very far into Sapolsky's research to realize that an alpha male baboon in a suit and tie could probably do a passable job of running a Wall Street firm or, in a black turtleneck, a Silicon Valley start-up. In fact, parallel research showed a parallel distribution of cortisol among British civil servants.

There are a couple of keys to this, and one is that stress is about control and the attempt of dominant players to exert control. But there is also a key point about chronic stress. In baboon society, aggressive behavior and punishment are an unrelenting way of life, or at least it was for these baboons. For a time. Sapolsky's research in Africa tracked a disease outbreak among the baboons that happened to be selective in its lethality to dominant males. After a critical mass of them died off, the surviving baboons reorganized without the violence and resulting cascade of cortisol. Peace prevailed. That is not to say that stress was removed from their lives—just that it was no longer the dominant force of their lives, and this is the refining point that brings us to Sapolsky's contribution at the 2005 conference.

Stress is one of those concepts that has been beaten to death in popular understanding, but the general discussion misses something important. The very mention of the word provokes something like the universal response to the mention of vampires in old horror movies: zero tolerance, and a sign of the cross to ward them off. The fact is, a complete absence of stress in your life is not an ideal state.

"For a short time, one or two hours, stress does wonderful things for the brain," Sapolsky told the conference. "More oxygen and glucose are delivered to the brain. The hippocampus, which is involved in memory, works better when you are stressed for a little while. Your brain releases more dopamine, which plays a role in the experience of pleasure, early on during stress; it feels wonderful, and your brain works better."

Dopamine is the big indicator here; it's the neurotransmitter wound up in our primary reward system, the big player in making us feel better and keeping us focused. The presence of dopamine signals something quite remarkable about stress. Sapolsky cited a bit of monkey research, simple and straightforward: researchers tracked dopamine when a monkey was given a reward each time it pressed a lever, and they compared the results with those when a monkey randomly got a reward only about half the time it pressed the lever. The results showed that the monkey released more dopamine in the latter case. More pleasure for half the number of rewards, but also when rewards are irregular or unexpected.

Sapolsky: "I said that lack of control is very stressful. Here a lack of control feels wonderful and your dopamine goes way up. What's the difference? As I mentioned earlier, the research shows that if your lack of control occurs in a setting that you perceive as malevolent and threatening, lack of control is a terrible stressor. If the lack of control occurs in a setting perceived as benign and safe, lack of control feels wonderful."

All of this is to say that our pleasure circuits are attuned to awareness and unexpected rewards, and stress is in this mix — not chronic unremitting stress that characterizes day-to-day life for many of us, but the ups and downs that flow from normal life. The pleasurable life is not stress-free, and Sapolsky argues that this realization provides a precise analogue for meditation:

> People think that you secrete stress hormones when there is stress, and when there is no stress, you don't secrete them or secrete just a little bit. You are at baseline. It was a long-standing tradition in the field to

consider the baseline to be extremely boring. What's now clear instead is that the baseline is a very active, focused, metaphorically muscular process of preparation for stress. The jargon used in the field is that it has permissible effect, allowing the stress response to be as optimal as possible. That's a wonderful endocrine analogue to the notion of meditation. A state of peace is not the absence of challenge. It is not the absence of alertness and energetic expenditure. If anything, it is a focusing of alertness in preparation. It absolutely matches the endocrine picture.

We think "alertness in preparation" is an exact summary of the hunter-gatherer state of mind, and now it appears that evolution has wired us to be rewarded by achieving it. Of course it has. The ideal state is not noise or absence of noise, stressed or relaxed, feast or famine, awake or asleep. This is more the case of defining one more edge between two states and then noting how our bodies are attuned to walking that line.

Cortisol can track this matter with stress, but there is a more interesting way that's emerging to gauge our undoing, our literal unraveling. Remember that confounding the issue of diseases of civilization was the unavoidable fact of nature that we all must die of something. Obviously, though, most of us would rather there be nothing more precise than "old age" written on the certificate under "cause of death." The process we'd all like to see in play (given the alternatives) is senescence, the unwinding of the biological clock spring.

The study of our DNA, though, has turned up an interesting measure of this process, structures called telomeres that serve as protective caps on the ends of strands of DNA. Telomeres seem to have some clear role in preserving the integrity of DNA through the countless divisions and recombinations that occur with cellular growth and reconstruction. They keep the code intact—but as we age, they seem to wear out, which is part of the reason the process of cellular growth becomes less reliable. And then we sag, sink, and wrinkle. Senescence.

Yet the decay of telomeres is not simply a chronological process, a measure of time, of old age. Besides time alone, conditions of our life can damage telomeres. And those conditions happen to be the ones we have been talking about throughout this book: bad nutrition, lack of sleep, flawed relationships, obesity, sedentary lives. All of this causes us to wear out before our time. Stress itself is now being tracked by telomere decay, just as it is with cortisol. So is lack of sleep, which brings real meaning to Worthman's contention that we pay for a lack of sleep in the currency of stress, as reported earlier.

This currency is denominated in telomerase, which is an enzyme the body secretes to protect telomeres. Dopamine may signal our sense of pleasure and well-being, but the presence of telomerase signals that we are not rushing our body's clock toward senescence. In 2010, one group of researchers published results that showed a significant increase in telomerase among participants in a meditation retreat.

BUILDING YOUR BRAIN

On this topic of meditation there is an interesting gap that pulls us back to the discussion of human evolution. But first, consider what is not going on in most forms of meditation. It is not about thinking; it's not what you think.

As you might imagine, years of tradition funneled through diverse cultures and personalities have created variations in the practice of meditation. The details differ, and in some traditions, practice actually does involve a sort of religious fixation on a specific object or person, like the Buddha. But more often than not, especially as the practice has been interpreted in Western tradition, in the austere forms of Zen Buddhism and in research labs, the actual focus of the mind during meditation involves pretty much nothing at all. One common approach is to simply sit and not try to control thoughts or sounds or the flow of events, but to observe and note the various streams that enter one's mind.

Another form of practice is more focused on a single set of sensations — more often than not the breath, or simply intense concentration on an imaginary point inside one's head, directly behind the eyes. Yet notice what is not happening in all of these practices. The practice itself is directed toward no particular goal or personality trait. Practitioners are not exercising the mind in mental acrobatics like memory drills, conundrums, or puzzle solving. They are certainly not instructing the center of self to become more moral, pious, or upright. One simply tries to quiet the background substrate in which thoughts flow.

In light of this, it seems somewhat odd that what we have reported does occur, that memory or performance or cognition or even physical health get better as a direct result of training the mind to do nothing. A demonstrated improvement in immune response from simply quieting the mind? Yes indeed. Or, more profound still, recent results from one research project show a link between meditation and increased brain mass, including increased gray matter in regions of the brain associated with learning, memory, and emotional regulation—the last linked to specific physical changes in the hippocampus and posterior cingulate regions of the brain.

What this is saying is that the brain responds to meditation as a muscle does to exercise, and of course it does. That was the implication from neuroscience's realization about neuroplasticity and neurogenesis. Yet it is wrong to say that meditation alone accomplishes a reshaping of the brain. The fact is, everything effects a reshaping of the brain, especially our relationships with one another. The tangible, weighable, measurable, energy-sucking organ is being built from the ground up, beginning even before we are born, and the whole stream of information we call life is doing the building work. The degree to which those relationships are healthy, especially when we are children, is the degree to which our brains are healthy.

What is different about meditation and a number of other practices like talk therapy or exercise or sound nutrition is that we are *deliberately* shaping our brains, intervening in the building process. Someone once argued that there is no choice about whether to train your dog. You either train your dog or your dog trains you. Something similar happens with our brains.

The new and urgent message, not just from meditation research but from neuroscience in general, is that we know now that directed forms of mental exercise begin shaping our brains in ways we want them to go. Davidson said in an online interview that what he has produced in his lab at Madison is really "the invitation to take more responsibility for our own brains. When we intentionally direct our minds in certain ways, that is literally sculpting the brain."

Yet this process is not completely independent from human design, which is to say what natural selection delivered us. Remember, meditation has no goal, but it is a sort of tune-up of the components. And yet from the process, a common thread emerges — a common end that is wholly in tune with our evolutionary history and hallmarks as a species.

Psychologists have devised a simple way of measuring this, a game that begins with giving volunteers real money, fifty bucks or so, and then placing them in a three-way relationship in which they dole out that money according to what other players do. And then, without the subjects knowing it, the testers rig the game so it appears as if one of the other players is stingy and is in fact punishing the third player by not doling out a fair share. The choice for the volunteer is whether to part with some of her own money to effect a more equitable distribution of the cash, and the test is real enough in that the volunteer, usually a broke undergrad, gets to keep whatever cash she has left after the game ends.

Davidson's lab has run this game on randomly selected subjects who undergo a short training in meditation, and after they do so, they give away more money. Researchers regard this as a measure of empathy. The meditative practice does not tell the subjects they should be more empathetic or equitable or compassionate or just. It does not offer skills for doing so. It simply quiets and tunes the mind. Once cleared of clutter, the mind reverts to its default mode set by evolution, which is empathy.

MINDFULNESS FOR EVERYONE

In psychological circles, Ellen Langer, a professor of psychology at Harvard, is known for bringing the term "mindfulness" into play. The term, of course, is much older in the English language, but Langer has secularized it, employed it as we have above in the more general hunter-gatherer state of mind. She is in fact known for a couple of experiments that bring this whole idea into common, general, no-nonsense experience. The first is the chambermaid experiment. She selected a sample of hotel chambermaids and asked them all whether they exercised. Most said they did not, although their work routines kept them active enough to meet the surgeon general's guidelines for healthy physical activity. Nonetheless, Langer recorded their body fat, waist-to-hip ratios, blood pressure, weight, and body mass index and then split the subjects into two groups. She followed around the members of one group through their daily routines and pointed out to them how the specific motions of their work looked like gym exercises. A month later, she interviewed everybody to make sure they had not changed behavior (like diet or exercise) and then redid the measurements. The group that had been told that their work resembled gym exercises in fact physically looked as though they had been exercising: they decreased their systolic blood pressure, weight, and waist-to-hip ratio, and they showed a 10 percent drop in blood pressure. The control group stayed the same. It appears that the mind literally can shape the body.

In a second famous experiment called "Counterclockwise,"

Langer rounded up a group of old men and housed them in quarters decorated and furnished as if it were twenty years earlier. The men began to look and act as if they were twenty years younger.

Langer has also recruited professional musicians and divided them into two groups, telling one to perform a piece to match their best-ever performance of that same piece. She told the other group to play a familiar piece in a new way, with subtle variations that only they would know. Then she had audiences evaluate the performances. The latter group of performers got higher marks from the audience. She then told salesmen to vary their pitch every time they gave it, instead of giving a rote presentation. They logged more sales as a result.

This last experiment steers us toward Langer's definition of mindfulness, and it is every bit as simple as "awareness." She doesn't teach subjects in her experiments how to meditate, but she does teach them how to "notice new things." That's all: notice new things. This is the same instruction that evolution issued to hunter-gatherers to ensure their survival.

Our favorite experiment in this vein was conducted not by Langer but by Daniel Simons of the University of Illinois at Urbana-Champaign and Christopher Chabris, at Harvard at the time of the research. In it they showed subjects an impromptu game of two teams passing a basketball back and forth. Subjects were asked to note how many times the basketball changed hands, meaning they were asked to pay attention to a single detail and account. Then, during the game, a guy in a gorilla suit walked onto the field of play and weaved among the players.

Remarkably, the participants in the experiment did not see

the gorilla. Not at all. They were too engaged in the counting, in the narrow task at hand.

Maybe Langer's instructions to be prepared for something new, for an anomaly, would have helped them see the gorilla in the room — but we think that any hunter-gatherer would have seen it, no problem.

7

Biophilia

Finding Our Better Nature in Nature

Now we need the great biologist E. O. Wilson and the idea of biophilia. (The term is widely attributed to Wilson but in fact traces to the German socialist philosopher and social psychologist Erich Fromm. He uses it much as Wilson does in the 1964 book *The Heart of Man*.) Wilson lays out the idea in deceptively simple terms: "Biophilia, if it exists, and I believe it exists, is the innately emotional affiliation of human beings to other living organisms. Innate means hereditary and hence part of ultimate human nature."

The real power of this idea is rooted in the implications of "innate." It means that it is encoded in us by evolution—and if it is programmed, then heeding that innate attraction has the power to ensure our well-being. There is something about the deep attachment to nature as opposed to attachment to the artificial world that confers fitness, or at least did confer fitness during most of the course of human evolution.

The logic of this is as follows: Humans, and all species, for that matter, succeed as a species only to the degree they are able to adapt to their environments. Humans, though, did this in part with big brains, by exercising a knowledge of the natural world—a task made more complex for our species by our varied habits and habitats and variety of diet, as we have already explored. Imagine for a moment how simple attentiveness to one's surroundings becomes when amplified with a bit of obsessiveness, of fascination, of real attachment—not merely observing but reveling in the conditions of nature. People with this trait would be more likely to survive. This is not to argue that there is a gene or a hormone for biophilia. Like most interesting traits in humans, this is far more likely a number of traits working together in a networked system. But it's easy enough to see how evolution might reward and amplify those traits. For example, an attraction to the color red causes one to notice it more, and in nature, red often equals ripe fruit.

And so it follows, as was the case with motion and running, protein and fats and sleep, that elements of our sense of well-being and happiness are wrapped up in this trait. This is a hypothesis we can take to the lab (and we will), but our first preferred venue for testing this idea is an ordinary scene. Most of us who have wandered forest trails, or even strolled urban parks, or even driven a scenic highway, can conjure this thought experiment. Think of the place in such a hike or drive where you stop to take it all in. On the highway, there will be a sign marking the "scenic turnout," a sign erected not because some highway engineer thought this was an opportune place to pull over but because so many people actually did pull over and the engineers needed to accommodate the demand. This tells us something in and of itself—but the parallel scene on a mountain trail tells us more. It often comes miles up the trail after winding through rock, scree, and trees, to a ridgetop and a grassy park with a sweeping view of a valley below, when a broad expanse of territory reveals itself—and then comes your urge to stop and take it in, to rest and settle with the peace of the place.

We brought you to this ordinary scene in the mountains for a reason. Look around for a moment—not to the panorama, but at your feet, on the ground. If you are in a place where mule deer or elk live, you will notice that this particular spot is littered with droppings. And just this spot. Everything you crossed en route was not so littered, despite the fact that the rest of your hike was an elk and deer habitat as well. This means simply that the elk bed here, spending sunny afternoons lounging and taking in the day. Those elk feces are hard evidence of our thesis, a deep kinship between you and those strange majestic animals, the sense that both of you have an innate preference for places like this because the vista makes you safe from predators and gives you vital knowledge of your surroundings. You can see, and you are safe. Evolution has written this in your programming for the same reasons it has written the same instructions in the program of elk. And for a moment in this place, animals do not know way more than you do. You read the signs the same as a wild elk does, and the signs say you are home.

This simple idea can translate into hard dollars and cents. Rooms with a view or houses fronted by a lake or stream replicate conditions important to us throughout evolution. Anthropologists who have studied bushmen invariably note that the nomadic wanderings of hunting and gathering are governed by daily cycles that place people in safe camps at night, always with access to water and with an unobstructed view of the surroundings. There is no reason for that preference to hold up millennia later other than a genetic memory—but an apartment with a commanding view of Central Park or waterfront property costs more. This is a measure of biophilia, the price tag on our genetically programmed preference for certain places.

The idea of biophilia has undergone rigorous testing, specifically the idea that we humans, just like any creature with a long history of serving as meat for predators, still seem to prefer vistas and fear enclosed spaces. There is, however, a flip side to this phenomenon that turns out to be just as telling: along with biophilia, there is a balancing set of predispositions tuned to our ancestral enemies. Besides preferences, we ought to have fears that are genetically encoded, biophobias, confirmed in a number of cross-cultural, controlled studies that show an innate aversion to creatures like spiders and snakes (especially snakes). These details are even more illuminating.

Some experiments do indeed show an innate fear of snakes, but in others researchers instead found what psychologists call "biologically prepared learning." That is, we seem to have pre-wired circuitry for learning some things better than others. We learn to fear spiders and snakes very quickly and retain the learning better than we retain other sorts of conditioning; this difference is most telling when compared with our learning about real hazards in the modern world.

Most of us today have far more reason to fear bare electrical wires or traffic than snakes, and yet researchers have found no innate aversion to or prepared learning about these, nor abilities to retain conditioned responses or learned experiences. This is in sharp contrast to the same sorts of experiences with spiders and snakes and fear of heights. Our modern world is full of hazards and pitfalls, and almost none of them are natural or anything like what our ancestors feared—and yet our minds dwell on the same fears that our ancestors had. A highway fatality now barely makes a headline, but a lethal grizzly bear attack gets page one play and is all the buzz on Twitter and Facebook the following day. All of which steers us toward an interesting conclusion.

"It suggests that when human beings remove themselves from the natural environment, the biophilic learning rules are not replaced by modern versions equally well adapted to artifacts," writes Wilson. "The brain evolved in a biocentric world, not a machine-regulated world. It would be therefore quite extraordinary to find that all learning rules related to that world have been erased in a few thousand years, even in the tiny minority of peoples who have existed for more than one or two generations in wholly urban environments."

Yet as a practical matter this offers enormous opportunity. Our attention to this topic is drawn not so much by vestigial fears of spiders and snakes; we are pursuing this idea because it points to some easily reachable antidotes and pathways, even literal pathways, and to our well-being in everyday life, urban and otherwise.

It's easy to see how society might have missed the importance of maintaining our ties to natural surroundings, and in fact there is research on this very issue. One study in particular demonstrates not only that contact with nature, something as simple as a walk in the park, makes us measurably better and a bit smarter but that the participants in the study underestimated the benefits. That is, the subjects tested better on some mental performance measures than they thought they would and didn't credit their walk in the park for the improvement.

The research was the work of the Canadian psychologists

Elizabeth K. Nisbet and John M. Zelenski, who wrote: "Modern lifestyles disconnect people from nature, and this may have adverse consequences for the well-being of both humans and the environment."

Their work fits within a larger body of research from around the world, and the net result of all of this is that we probably can remove the qualifier "may" from the above statement.

When we deny these preferences, these innate attachments to nature, we suffer, and this is a big part of what ails us in a high-tech world of artifice that's increasingly disconnected from nature. The author Richard Louv has argued that this is a key affliction of civilization, even going so far as to give it a name: nature deficit disorder. Louv built his case on ten years' worth of interviews with parents in the United States and concluded that the glitzy attractions of the virtual world, coupled with what he cites as oversensationalized media coverage about the dangers of the outdoors, have created an epidemic of detachment from nature among modern children and, by extension, adults.

This is troubling enough, even on the obvious level that nature contains all of biological life, and children ought to gain the knowledge and appreciation on offer in the wild. But Louv and others point out that there are more subtle issues, and those parallel some we have already talked about in detailing the afflictions of civilization. To cite a few, play in nature exposes kids (and everyone else) to a full range of microbes to support their internal microbiomes and challenge and tune their immune systems; these microbes also fight autoimmune disease, the epidemic of absence. Also, play outdoors exposes people to the full spectrum of light, with a variety of benefits, not the least among them regulating melatonin and sleep cycles but also making for healthy levels of vitamin D. Shortage of vitamin D is an epidemic in its own right, but in this light, it is also a subset of the epidemic of nature deficit disorder.

All of this goes a long way to explain why we are evolved to be in nature, and therefore to value it. All of this supports the hypothesis of biophilia.

Much of this line of thought began in the late 1970s in Ann Arbor, an appropriate center of origin given that its very name includes a reference to trees. While working on his PhD in geography, Roger S. Ulrich happened to notice that Ann Arborites on their way to a mall had a habit of driving out of their way to avoid a freeway and instead took a tree-lined route. That began a series of research projects to demonstrate that these people were in fact deriving some benefit from the eccentric (and more costly) route. Ulrich used an EEG to measure alpha wave activity in research subjects. Alpha waves are associated with serotonin production, and serotonin counters depression. Natural scenes and association with nature did indeed show positive results with alpha waves, and both also had a positive effect against anxiety, anger, and aggression.

In their 2012 book, *Your Brain on Nature: The Science of Nature's Influence on Your Health, Happiness, and Vitality*, the authors Eva M. Selhub, a medical doctor, and Alan C. Logan, a naturopath, summarize Ulrich's work along with examples from around the world. Among them: subjects in an adult care center in Texas showed decreased cortisol levels (the stress hormone) when in a garden setting; a study in Kansas using EEG showed less stress in subjects when plants were in the room; researchers in Taiwan, using measures like EEGs and skin conductance, noted therapeutic effects in subjects viewing streams, valleys, rivers, terraces, water, orchards, and farms; 119 research subjects in Japan showed less stress response when transplanting plants in pots than they did when simply filling pots with soil; and another group of subjects in Japan had lower heart rates after viewing natural scenes for twenty minutes.

Japan, in fact, is the center of some of the most interesting and innovative thinking about this issue; the research has been formalized through the Japanese Society of Forest Medicine and a national movement called *shinrin-yoku*, which translates poorly into English but means something like bathing or basking in the forest. The movement has spawned a series of studies that use objective markers like cortisol, heart rate, and blood pressure to demonstrate that there are real and measurable benefits to well-being and mental performance through simple contact with nature. For instance, a number of studies have shown that people in hospitals get better measurably faster if they are in a room with a window or have a bit of green as simple as a potted plant. Placing potted plants in view of workers at one factory reduced time lost to sick leave by 40 percent.

One of the more interesting findings in the Japanese research is a sort of Goldilocks effect that shows up with trees and potted plants, and results have been replicated elsewhere. It seems there is a sweet spot. Up until that point, benefits to one's well-being increase when more plants or trees are introduced to a room — but beyond the sweet spot, subjects begin to feel worse. Too many plants or trees, and we begin to feel uneasy. The herd of elk we visited earlier could predict this response. It replicates our ease with open views but relative unease in overdense forests, where we and elk were more vulnerable to predators in evolutionary times. The dense forest, as Dorothy and her friends understood, was the habitat of lions and tigers and bears — even in Oz.

Taken together, these findings begin to offer some advice for public policy and design. That is, greenways, open space, land-scaping, and even potted plants ought to be integrated into any efficient design of urban space as a simple, cost-effective invest-ment in public health and tranquility. Research in both schools and workplaces has demonstrated clearly that performance of students and workers increases as a result of these simple, low-cost, and uncontroversial measures.

Japan leads not only in research into the tangible benefits of exposure to nature but also in the commitment to making it happen. The government has already invested $4 million in research and over the past ten years has launched one hundred forest therapy centers around the country. The movement is tak-ing root throughout Asia, with active research in Taiwan and Korea. The government of South Korea is spending $140 million on a forest therapy center.

But where this becomes really interesting is in more costly matters like health care, and indeed some of the more sophisti-cated research has demonstrated that death rates from diseases like cancer decline in areas with more forest cover. Researchers used GIS (geographic information system) mapping tools to control for all other factors, like smoking and socioeconomic sta-tus, and found that the dominance of forests alone decreased death rates from cancer. This macro-level series of investigations gets support from individual research that demonstrates a posi-tive immune response from natural settings. Demonstrably and measurably, simple exposure to nature makes you more resistant to disease.

A study in the Netherlands examined the records of 195 doctors who served a total of 345,143 patients. Researchers were looking for a correlation between living near green space and the rate of morbidity, or being sick. They found rates lower for fifteen of twenty-four diseases examined for those people living within a kilometer of green space, and the relationship was especially important for poorer people. The benefits of green space were strongest for those with anxiety disorders and depression.

Yet as Nisbet noted in individual subjects — even subjects getting the direct benefit of this exposure — people fail to appreciate the value of green space, which is likely an enormous factor in why this is also underappreciated in public policy. But the fine details of our cluelessness on this topic become even more interesting and suggest that there is far more to this than we might think. Some of the research with biophobia of spiders and snakes, for instance, used subliminal exposure to pictures of the creepy crawlers. Participants were shown video of some innocuous scenes, and researchers slipped in a picture of a snake that was not really visible — it was present for only a few milliseconds, passing too fast to be comprehended. Yet there was still a fear response. And there wasn't a parallel response to subliminal exposure to more modern hazards like bare electrical wires. At least in this experiment, nature was having a measurable effect on subjects' emotional states, and the subjects had no idea why.

This lack of perception is even more interesting as seen in some work done with *shinrin-yoku* in Japan that looked at aromas in the forests. Trees and other plants exude literally scores of phytochemicals that make their way to our olfactory system, which provides a direct pathway to the brain. The class of chemicals involved are called phytoncides, and many of them have profound effects on the brain, such as lowering stress hormones, regulating pain, and reducing anxiety. Notably, some of them up-regulate powerful tools in our immune systems called natural killer cells, first-line defensive weapons against infections like influenza and common colds. Yet many of these phytoncides are undetectable as aromas. We have no idea that a natural setting is chemically stimulating our immune systems as we simply inhale the open air.

Interestingly, the Japanese research showed that this increased immune response endured. A group of Japanese businessmen who were the research subjects showed a 40 percent increase in natural killer cells after a walk in the woods, but follow-up research showed that their killer cells were still elevated by 15 percent over baseline a month later.

Yet by now, you may be noticing that there's something else in the air, that the pathways and effects of nature parallel those we talked about with sleep, exercise, nutrition, and even meditation. There's more to this. As with these other topics, researchers have begun to use fMRIs in their research; as a result, they have found where exactly it is that nature works in our brains, even pinpointing it as specifically as the parahippocampal gyrus, which is an area rich in opioid receptors (special cells for attaching to opioids, a family of chemicals that includes drugs like morphine and has powerful effects on the brain).

"This was an incredible finding, revealing that nature is like a little drop of morphine for the brain," write Selhub and Logan.

Korean researchers took this a step further and found that urban settings activated a brain area associated with anger and depression, but that natural scenes produced a pronounced effect in the anterior cingulate and insula. This is an important center for empathy, and the effect was confirmed through psychological tests in which people are asked to give away money to other people, exactly as was the case with the meditation studies we cited. And just as with meditation, there was no goal or described pathway for becoming a more empathetic person. Just as the simple act of calming one's brain made one more empathetic, so did a simple walk in the woods.

All of this research seems to be steering us to an almost mystical aspect of biophilia because we are dealing with the unseen and unperceived. Yet it is not mystical or supernatural—just real physical forces we have no ability to perceive (or maybe our urban ways have deprived us of the ability to perceive them). Maybe this is what so fascinates and engages hunter-gatherers or the Koyukon people we spoke of in the last chapter. Maybe they are so engaged with the natural world because the conditions of their lives have trained their minds to see and comprehend the gorilla in the room, a real presence that pulls them in and makes them happy. We mean to leave this possibility open for you to explore.

But at the same time, know that there is plenty of hard evidence that these unseen forces make a real and measurable difference in our lives, and we need not go as far afield as invisible, unsmellable phytochemicals to make the point. We also don't perceive the ultraviolet B wavelengths of light that cause our skin to manufacture vitamin D. But it is nonetheless a fact that full body exposure to sunlight for thirty minutes causes your skin to manufacture ten thousand to twenty thousand IUs of vitamin D, and it is an understatement to say that your body needs vitamin D. Your body *must* have it or you will get sick.

As we said, vitamin D deficiency is a growing problem among modern people. One nutritionist we interviewed was performing blood tests on poor inner-city children in Boston, and we thought that conversation would steer us toward talk of blood glucose and diabetes. It did. But the same nutritionist was equally alarmed by the vitamin D deficiency she found in these children. Michael Holick, an expert on vitamin D at Boston University School of Medicine, told the *New York Times* that on average, Caucasian Americans are short of ideal levels of vitamin D by about a third, and African Americans by about half. And many individuals are much worse off.

In severe cases in children, this deficiency can lead to the disease rickets. But in both children and adults, lack of vitamin D can lead to increased risk of colon, breast, and prostate cancer; high blood pressure and heart disease; osteoarthritis; and autoimmune disorders. We think all of this can be headed off by simply spending more time outdoors, in the sun, which is by far the most direct way to solve this deficiency.

Yet what is intriguing about this topic of nature is the way it seems to double back on all else we have talked about so far, so that we begin talking about our place in nature and then high blood pressure, lack of movement, autoimmune disorders, and depression all come into play. We can take this a couple of steps further. The researchers S. C. Gominak and W. E. Stumpf published a paper detailing the results of treating insomnia with vitamin D after sleep doctors noticed that some of their patients who just happened to be taking vitamin D supplements saw improvement in their sleep patterns. That led to a two-year study of fifteen hundred patients with all sorts of sleep disorders, which showed that areas of the brain with important vitamin D receptors also happened to be areas involved in allowing a positive result for the patients in the trial: sleep.

The researchers concluded: "We propose the hypothesis that sleep disorders have become epidemic because of widespread vitamin D deficiency."

Here's another crossover: remember the hygiene hypothesis—that modern people, especially urban people, are showing a rapid increase in autoimmune diseases simply because they live in a sanitized, built environment and so have removed their immune systems from the challenges of the real world? We evolved living in contact with and dealing with the full complement of microbes, and when removed from that contact, we suffer the results, especially in our internal biome. To be healthy, our internal ecosystems need to be connected to external ecosystems. We connect them by spending time outdoors, in nature, away from sterile, artificial environments.

To be sure, there are layers and complexities to this issue beyond most of our understanding (we think some even beyond all of our comprehension), but the prescription here need not be complicated. For instance, we have long been advocates of connecting children with the natural world by ensuring that they get outdoors, dig in the dirt, and bask in the sun. The research bears out this prescription, and besides that, it sounds like fun.

ANOTHER LEVER

At the very least, these findings suggest some direction for public policy on such matters as greenways, trail systems, and open space, but we hope they also suggest possibilities for your own life. If a simple walk in the woods accomplishes this much alone, what about combining these benefits? What about meditation in a natural setting, or attending to nutrition and taking daily walks along the stream—and adding an adequate amount of high-quality sleep to the mix? All along, we have built the case for re-wilding your life. It almost goes without saying that part of the process ought to be some real, physical contact with things wild.

And if a potted plant helps us inside, are trees better help outside? How far up the mountain can one go? Do I really want to run on a treadmill in the middle of a gym lined with television monitors and smelling of, well, not trees and flowers? And might there be an advantage to running instead in the mountains, to movement in nature, which Selhub and Logan call "exercise squared"?

As we progress in our story, the lever effect is going to come increasingly into play. Remember the lever? Beverly Tatum gave it that name when she talked about sleep, that the simple act of getting more sleep made her attentive to other matters, like nutrition and exercise. One thing led to another. In the authors' lives, this matter of contact with nature is also a lever, and one with a profound effect. A lot of this comes together at Rancho La Puerta. That's where we met Tatum, but also the remarkable Deborah Szekely, now in her nineties, who cofounded the ranch in the 1940s. She also founded and is pressing forth with her project Wellness Warrior, to do the sort of grassroots change necessary to fundamentally rework society. The message is fitness and nutrition, but the lever that works these is contact with nature, a conscious goal of re-wilding the people, sometimes rich and famous, who are the ranch's clients. Szekely says everything begins with the mountain at Rancho La Puerta, which is another way of saying everything begins with nature. Szekely and the ranch loom large in John Ratey's own story, and we will get to that in time.

THE JOYS OF ADVERSITY

You might be thinking that nature can be capricious and cruel, and that maybe it's better to stick to the gym. But we think this capriciousness is a part of the real benefit of living as much of your life as you can in wild settings.

The romanticism of nature means that it conjures birds singing and warm rays of sunshine shafting through trees on a sunny afternoon—a Disney version ready to embrace us with warm, open arms. This is not nature, but, more to the point, we would not reap all of these rewards from our contact with nature if it were. And this realization brings us again to the slippery slope of evolutionary arguments that cohere too tightly to our assumptions about the crown of creation, when we think that nature somehow had us in mind through its billions of years of unfathomable motion, or that nature has our best interests at heart and will mother us. To quote the evolutionary biologist Richard Dawkins, "Nature is not cruel, only pitilessly indifferent. This is one of the hardest lessons for humans to learn. We cannot admit that things might be neither good nor evil, neither cruel nor kind but simply callous—indifferent to all suffering, lacking all purpose."

And this is indifference we need. Robert Sapolsky's baboons headed us in exactly this direction when we first met them a chapter ago, with the vital and unexpected realization that predictable rewards failed to fully stimulate the brain's circuitry of rewards, and that it was only when researchers removed the regularity that the brains lit up in happiness. Nature does not rig the game in our favor, and so it would follow that our brains and our happiness had to evolve to match an unrigged game.

At the same time, this lack of regularity demands our awareness. Our attention makes our lives better by stimulating mindfulness. And we have seen this in action, even before the monkeys. Remember when we went for a run with our dog along a mountain path? You probably realized then and should realize now that the natural setting was in fact the key element of that activity, the major player—that and the full engagement of your brain in complex and varied motion. When we first introduced the scene, we were making a point about variability and the simple physical mechanics of motion. That is, the undulating terrain and capricious weather of a mountain run deliver the random ups and downs, obstacles and challenges to recruit a wide variety of muscles and motions. This is what the body evolved to expect and what best stimulates the brain as it coordinates the body's physical motions. But there is not a clear line between the variability provided by nature and the larger connections we are making now. The environment randomly dealt out a set of mental challenges, some of them with real consequences, like a stumble, a broken ankle, a cliff, a snow squall, or a bear.

Trail running is an odd sport, and we are not arguing that everybody ought to do it—but we come back to it because it illustrates some of the seminal ideas of the book. We have every reason to expect these runners to be just another bunch of jocks, with opinions and sentiments much like those of Olympic marathoners, bikers, weight lifters, or soccer players. But there are some intriguing differences in behavior that we think are relevant to our larger points. We think these differences stem in part from the natural context and evolutionary precedent of this activity.

First, the sport is growing faster than probably any other. *UltraRunning* magazine reports that 63,530 runners finished ultramarathons in 2012, ultramarathons defined as any distance greater than the 26.2 miles of a marathon but almost exclusively run on trails on mountains and in deserts and forests. That number represents a 22 percent increase over the year before but a more than twentyfold increase over 1980. But further, this is not just a sport for young studs bursting with testosterone. The sport is reasonably gender-balanced, and some races are won by women. And there are big-time major event winners in their forties and active participants in their sixties and seventies, senior citizens finishing hundred-mile events. We think all of this enthusiasm stems from the fact that the sport seems to closely resemble what we did in our evolutionary past. The basic elements of mountain running appeal to those deeply seated urges encoded in us by evolution.

All of this, it turns out, has produced an interesting internal conversation, and it is worth eavesdropping on the blogs and websites. For example, take this post from Willie McBride from the popular website for trail runners iRunFar, built, remarkably, from ideas from Erich Fromm, the German philosopher we credited at the start of the chapter with the term "biophilia." McBride was pondering his seemingly contradictory attachment to social media on the one hand and mountain wilderness on the other:

Our need for experiencing both the rawest nature and the most instantaneous social technologies may seem contradictory but the root cause of these peculiar rituals stems from a deep and basic desire. We want to be connected, to be a part of something bigger than our individual selves.

In *The Art of Loving*, Erich Fromm writes, "The human race in its infancy still feels one with nature. The soil, the animals, the plants are still man's world. He identifies himself with animals.... But the more the human race emerges from these primary bonds, the more it separates itself from the natural world, the more intense becomes the need to find new ways of escaping separateness."

Fromm further believed that this devastating departure from nature is the root cause of all human suffering: "The experience of separation arouses anxiety. It is indeed the source of all anxiety. Being separate means being cut off, without any capacity to use my human powers. Hence, to be separate means to be helpless, unable to grasp the world, things and people actively. It means that the world can invade me without my ability to react."

And so this idea begins with nature and our need for connection with nature, as we have argued, because of its indifference. But the flip side of this is just as interesting and is implicit in our need for connection. In a perfect world, we face nature's indifference by connecting and drawing support from people who are not indifferent.

8

Tribe

The Molecule That Binds Us to One Another

We have been saving this story, one of our favorites, until now. It is odd that the research behind this story existed at all. It was examining a truly weird question about the safety of mothers sleeping with infants—weird because, through most of human history and in most contemporary societies, even, no one would question the safety of mothers sleeping with infants. There was, however, a particular focus of this experiment having to do with the relative positions of the two bodies being studied. Science has determined that there is a specific arrangement that does indeed optimize safety, a way for mother to curl around baby that makes the whole situation pretty bombproof, so that mother won't roll onto baby and hurt her. This was the fear that originally prompted the research.

Remember the example we cited early in this book about a dog having a litter of pups? The dog seemed to know all the proper steps of the process without instruction. Same deal with mothers sleeping with infants, or at least some mothers. The researchers found that mothers who were breastfeeding their infants assumed the prescribed position of maximum safety without instruction — even first-time mothers. Mothers who were not breastfeeding did not.

The dominant hormones of childbirth and lactation are prolactin and oxytocin, and it is this latter thread we pick up now. No better place to begin than at the very beginning, each of our literal beginnings, because this is the core relationship of human society and behavior, the one that explains who we are. True enough, oxytocin figures prominently in childbirth and lactation, but it continues to exert profound influences throughout our lives.

MOVING WITH OTHERS

At one point in thinking about this book, it occurred to us we were missing an important piece of our story, and we realized that Eva Selhub might be able to tell us what that was. The hunch came from a personal observation. We had followed Selhub's work and had spoken with her and her coauthor, Alan C. Logan, about their book, *Your Brain on Nature*, which provided a great deal of the information about biophilia in our last chapter. Beyond this, though, Selhub is a conventionally trained medical doctor who quickly moved beyond that training to study the healing power of nature, nutrition, and exercise, as well as meditation and traditional practices of healing, such as qigong. Her practice has followed many of the paths we have traced in this book, yet during our initial meeting with her, we couldn't help but notice that she was onto something new, that personally she had hit a stride that had pumped a fresh level of physical and mental vitality into her life. We wanted to know what it was.

And so we sat for a pleasant hour's conversation one sunny afternoon in Boston, and Selhub began by confirming our observations that in recent months she had in fact become a "very different person." She told us that the proximate cause of this was simple enough—deceptively so. She had joined a CrossFit gym, the regimen of physical exercise we spoke about earlier, with movements designed to provide a wide variety of challenges and ranges of motion that the human body probably encountered throughout evolutionary time. Yet this new variety of movement was not the whole story. It was certainly part of the explanation, but something else was at work, and that's mostly what Selhub wanted to talk about during our conversation.

Selhub admitted up front to a deep-seated loathing of gyms and the conditioned flee response to competitive athletics that's adopted by too many kids thanks to ill-conceived physical education programs. In her telling, the real attraction in her Cross-Fit practice was community.

"It feels good to have the rewards, to not only be able to excel and do something you've never been able to do but to compete with other people and have them be excited for you. For me, if it was just the competition, it wouldn't work, but it's the community. It's the camaraderie," she told us. "It's really a community.... It's kids running around, seeing parents and adults exercise and do crazy things, hugging, laughing, talking. It feels like the way it is supposed to be."

Feels like it is supposed to be.

Return for a second to the record compiled by Elizabeth

Marshall Thomas of her family's experience living among the Ju/wasi people of the Kalahari Desert in the 1950s. She quotes her mother, who wrote extensively about the experience:

> The [Ju/wasi] are extremely dependent emotionally on the sense of belonging and companionship.... Separation and loneliness are unendurable to them. I believe their wanting to belong and be near is actually visible in the way families cluster together in an encampment and in the way they sit huddled together, often touching someone, shoulder against shoulder, ankle across ankle. Security and comfort for them lie in their belonging to their group free from the threat of rejection and hostility.

Tribalism is a cultural universal, so identified by paleoanthropologists as one of the salient characteristics that has defined humanity since the beginning. The intense bonding of *Homo sapiens* was likely a major factor, if not *the* major factor, in giving us the edge that made us the lone survivor in our line of upright bipedal apes. Literally, we can trace our bonds in our bones, but better still to trace it in oxytocin, a chemical that's not just about nursing mothers. All women have it. So do all men. It holds us together. We're using oxytocin here to build the case that your well-being depends on solid relationships with other people.

THE BONDING AGENT

Sue Carter is at sea for a few minutes trying to decide where to begin, an excusable bit of indecision. How does one begin to summarize forty years of research into the effects of a single molecule, let alone one that's front and center at the core of human behavior (and the behavior of other species)? Evolution has been leaning on oxytocin and its close chemical relatives, especially vasopressin, to perform a variety of vital functions for a very long time, predating even humans but also predating mammals— even stretching back to the unimaginably distant and dank recesses of the evolutionary tunnel when vertebrates first split from the simpler creatures without spines. Vasopressin is an ancient chemical that likely appeared when all of life was contained in a water world, making it necessary to regulate the flow of water from inside to out of the organisms. It still does that job, even among the terrestrials, including humans.

Carter was also jet-lagged, having flown home the day before from Morocco, but she nonetheless had agreed to a conversation in her new town house just outside Chapel Hill, North Carolina, where she recently moved her work after spending most of her career as a neurobiologist at the University of Chicago. She takes a spot on a comfortable couch and is quickly joined by her Chin, a Japanese spaniel lapdog. And then she decides to begin where her work began in the 1970s: with prairie voles, an innocuous and silent mouselike species that navigates the tangled plant world of North American grassland ecosystems, mostly unseen by all except owls and biologists.

She began working in association with the field biologists who were asking the questions common in that discipline in the 1970s, questions that mostly had to do with survival and crashing population—and, when evolutionary ideas came into the picture, with the physical makeup of the beast in question, because then the emphasis was on finding those physical attributes that conferred fitness. At that time, prairie voles were undergoing boom-and-bust cycles—population explosions followed by crashes; it's the sort of phenomenon that alarmed biologists then but is now better understood as the normal course of events, especially among ground-level rodents. But the researchers quickly came to understand that there was something truly odd about this obscure little species of rodent. They were social. There was a vibrant vole society, and holding it together was monogamy (or at least that's how it looked from a hawk's-eye view), strong pair bonds between a single male and a single female, which is an uncommon practice among mammals.

What is most curious about this is that meadow voles—a closely related but separate species, the same genus in the same habitat—are not monogamous. All but a trained biologist— even owls—would be hard-pressed to spot the difference between a prairie vole and a meadow vole, yet prairie voles go in for life-long bonding to a single mate and meadow voles do not. In the '70s monogamy was thought to be a complex, evolved behavior like bipedalism or omnivory, and so followed an evolutionary line and logic in a predictable progression. But here it was, a distinctive behavior dropped into a single species without warning, like a plug-in option in a new model year of a car.

Back then, though, evolutionary biologists had a ready explanation for monogamy, rare as it was in mammals—an explanation based in sexual selection. That is, a male bonds to a given female and invests his energy in raising the young because they are his genetic issue. This in turn is rooted in the idea of what is famously labeled the "selfish gene," meaning that evolution selects for genes that perpetuate themselves and so selects for individuals that ensure perpetuation of their own genes over those of others. This, for instance, is the common explanation for the widespread practice of infanticide in the animal world, including among human animals: males, on encountering a new female, often kill her young so that they might replace them with their own genetic issue. In most cultures, including ours, death rates among children with stepfathers are about equal to those among other mammals.

Even in her early work, though, Carter was skeptical of this explanation for monogamy in prairie voles. "I had been exposed to enough sociobiology and evolutionary biology to assume that reproduction was the core of evolutionary theory. I don't think it is true. I think it is actually social interactions that are driving many aspects of behavior," she told us.

She was right, but it was not until the 1980s and the availability of certain tools for analyzing DNA that the fuller story emerged. Monogamous in outward appearances these prairie voles might be, but the undeniable evidence of the genes of vole pups demonstrated that these loyal males laboring their lives away raising pups were in fact cuckolds. About half of the pups were not their genetic issue. What's more, this rough ratio held up across the animal kingdom, especially among birds, for which monogamy is far more common. Depending on whom you ask and when, you will likely as not be told that humans are monogamous, but if you ask DNA about this, the story is much the same as for other animals. Sexually monogamous? Well, no. Voles and all the rest of the animals prefer marriage of convenience, which does not mean that the concept of monogamy is irrelevant, but it does need refining. It does not describe a sexual behavior, an adaptation based in reproduction. Rather, it describes a social adaptation that is indeed useful in ensuring a next generation, even a selfish gene generation. Half of the kids might not be the kin of papa vole, but half of them are, and stable social arrangements make everybody better off.

Yet this realization meant that the inquiry had wandered into what was then shaky ground for biologists, who were used to considering issues like prey base, carrying capacity, length of stride, and length of fang. Monogamy was not a physical attribute; it was a behavior. But the evidence was saying that the behavior was innate, not learned. But more to the point, vole society started to uncannily resemble that of humans, and no one really had any idea where that came from.

"They have a social system that looks like humans': long-lasting pair bonds, two parents taking care of young, incest avoidance, extended families—just about everything that is cardinal to human society," Carter said.

But not all of them, and not all of their lives. There are a couple of modes of prairie vole living, and all of this talk of sex completely ignores something important: those voles that ignore sex. This is a common thread in all social animals, even termites and ants. We have long wondered why so many members of, say, a bee colony are simply not players in reproduction, that task being relegated to the few fertile: a queen and the several drones who are her mates. Most bees go through life oblivious to mating, and it is not that different with voles. Most of these rodents spend life in what Carter labeled a "prepubertal" stage. But biologists soon discovered what flipped that switch: a simple matter of a timely meeting with an appropriate mate. Each half of the budding couple discovers the other by chance while they are still in that prepubertal state, but the encounter itself triggers a response in each that looks very much like going through puberty. The male especially is completely transformed in a matter of hours from a clueless, sexless naïf to a rather fiercely attached partner, and the partnership lasts for life. At the root of this transformation, Carter figured out, was oxytocin and, especially in the male, vasopressin. These are two closely related biochemicals, technically neuropeptides (brain chemicals). This discovery alone ratchets up the relevance of the finding to the human condition: oxytocin is the most common gene-generated molecule in the human brain. In voles, it is the transformative switch.

And not just in prairie voles, it turns out, and this is in many ways the finding that nailed the centrality of this single molecule in the foundational behavior of a whole series of widely unrelated species. That initial work with prairie voles has spawned what Carter characterizes today as a "tsunami" of research. Literally hundreds of labs worldwide are working on this single molecule, but one of the early eureka experiments involved giving oxytocin to species such as rats. Males of this species are not given to hanging around rearing young and helping out with the housework. These males are by nature more inclined to be, well, rats—but oxytocin-dosed rats adopted monogamous habits, including attentive pup rearing. Even in the close relative of prairie voles, the meadow voles, tweaking their brains to enhance their ability to feel the effects of oxytocin caused exactly the same behavioral shift.

The initial research about oxytocin predated the work on voles. As early as the 1950s, the neuropeptide had been identified and cited for its role in birth, lactation, and even sexual attraction. Further work in sheep and rats in the 1970s showed oxytocin's role in bonding between mothers and young rats and sheep. Yet demonstrating oxytocin's ability to organize the social system of prairie voles has tipped off scientists to roles for this single molecule far beyond the fundamentals of intercourse and reproduction.

It is the social molecule, and interest in it has built to something of a fever pitch with the realization that, although the molecule is manufactured deep in the brain and has its most profound effects there, it need not be injected directly into the brain, as was painstakingly done in the early research. It works its magic administered as a simple nasal spray, which is by far the most direct route to the brain, as cocaine users know. Some substances that we inhale quickly enter the brain, as we talked about with the aromas of nature in the last chapter.

As a practical matter, this has made the experiment with human subjects easier and a lot less invasive, ramping up this line of inquiry. Notably, experiments using standard tests for altruism, exactly like those we saw with meditation and exposure to nature, have delivered clear demonstrations that oxytocin enhances empathy and altruism. Oxytocin made subjects more likely to part with their money to offset what they saw as unfairness to another person. Oxytocin also enhances what psychologists call social cognition—that is, social skills. For instance, we can easily see how—and research has demonstrated this— our social bonds are dependent on our brain's ability to recognize faces, and oxytocin enhances that ability. It also enhances the ability to identify emotional states as they are displayed on faces, meaning the ability to read emotions in others. A whole series of experiments has shown the molecule's ability to enhance trust in others, and this idea expands how we might think about the importance of social relationships.

Research has also shown that oxytocin plays a key role in business transactions, especially in establishing trust. This is not as squishy as it might sound. Economists will tell you that the workings of the marketplace depend on a foundation of trust, that the glue of our economic lives rests on our ability to trust one another well enough to do deals. Follow this idea backward now through evolutionary time, and you can begin to see where this winds through the human condition, and how this group cohesion is part of our evolutionary success, our ability to adapt and prosper. Trust enables economy, a rule best demonstrated in negative examples, in places where anarchy and chaos have undermined all trust. Those places have little hope of economic development.

There are a couple of interesting asides in this same line of research. People engaged in business transactions produce a spurt of oxytocin. If one person gives another person ten dollars, the recipient's oxytocin levels spike a bit. But here's the kicker: if a computer gives that same person ten dollars, his levels of oxytocin do not increase. And there's a bit of intraspecific research that is our personal favorite: if you engage your dog, your oxytocin level increases, as you might expect — but your dog's oxytocin level increases even more.

Take these realizations together, and it's easy to see how some of them might provoke a scientific feeding frenzy. You can get a hint of this in the appearance of a recent popular book about oxytocin that's gushing with promise and titled *The Moral Molecule*. This chemical begins to look like a magic bullet, especially to people with autism. Remember, autism is characterized by that very lack of social ability that seems at the center of oxytocin's field of expertise. Things like enhancing the ability to recognize facial cues and other such social skills can seem like exactly what the doctor might order, and, in fact, some work has been done with autistic people that encourages this conclusion. So here appears an inviting target right up the center of the medical model's line of thinking: an easily synthesized molecule that can be administered in a simple nasal spray, is already the most common molecule in the human brain, and deals straight on with one of modern medicine's most intractable maladies— and at the same time spins off into trust, empathy, love, and understanding. What's not to love? What's not to love for Big Pharma?

Science magazine caught this drift in an article in January 2013 that began as follows:

> Few substances produced by the human body have inspired as much hoopla as oxytocin. Recent newspaper articles have credited this hormone with promoting the kind of teamwork that wins World Cup soccer championships and suggested that supplements of the peptide could have prevented the dalliances and subsequent downfall of a certain high ranking U.S. intelligence official. Although the breathless media coverage often goes too far, it reflects a genuine and infectious excitement among many scientists about the hormone's role in social behavior.

Well, maybe, but haven't we been down this road before, seen the allure of magic-bullet, single-pathway solutions?

Or as Carter put it: "The public wants a fast answer. If we know it works, why don't we make a drug out of it [oxytocin]?"

She added that such a solution "seems a bit arrogant and stupid."

To begin with, we've known from the very beginning of the work on voles that if you focus on the yin of oxytocin and ignore the yang of vasopressin, you are going to miss some key elements. And, in fact, yin-yang probably overstates the separation, because both neuropeptides are very closely related in function, chemical structure, and evolutionary history. Both are important to both genders, but vasopressin has a decidedly male skew.

This is probably more than an interesting aside because everything in the human body is connected, but vasopressin research also appears in a very different arena, one that explores its function as a regulator for water. In its finer points, however, this regulation by vasopressin (which is in its chemical structure almost identical to oxytocin) turns out to be far more interesting and, in fact, seminal to some of our earlier discussions about exercise. Vasopressin is what gave us the ability to practice the form of persistence hunting that David Carrier (the mountain runner–researcher at the University of Utah) talked about and what helped him begin to understand why humans were born to run. We developed this skill in an arid landscape, after all. Modern bushmen still do persistence hunting in the desert, and observers have noticed that they do it without drinking water. Thomas, in fact, noted that groups of men who hunt and women who go on daylong forays of gathering food take nothing more than an ostrich eggshell full of water to last the whole day under a desert sun. That is to say, these bushmen could run full days in scorching heat on an amount of water that some people advise modern runners to drink every half hour.

The South African researcher Tim Noakes has done an

extensive study of this matter and has shown pretty clearly that the more excessive modern advice on runners and water is, in fact, just that: excessive. The data show that the advice to drink lots of water (actually to "hydrate," and that's part of the problem — that we no longer drink water; we "hydrate") is simply wrong. Noakes's analysis showed that runners who were the most dehydrated after marathon-length races actually tended to win. More to the point, no one suffered medical problems from dehydration, while those who drank the recommended amount of water or sports drinks often suffered severe consequences from *too much* water. Some even died.

The deal is, exercise, especially running in hot conditions, triggers a cascade of vasopressin, which causes the runner's body to conserve water. That's the very trick that allowed the bushmen to succeed in the desert, and the deaths in modern-day marathons are the result of our thinking that we need a solution like "hydration" to overrule evolution's design. One more example.

But the more telling bit of information in this aside is evidence that both vasopressin, as we have shown, and oxytocin, the "social molecule" we are trying to bottle in nasal sprayers, are triggered by exercise. Chalk up one more brain benefit from exercise. And by now, it should be no surprise that running, movement, social bonding, and emotional well-being have a common chemical pathway. Chemically, these seemingly disparate topics hang together, and we ought to pay attention to that as a big signpost of evolution's design.

But back to the social side of this chemistry. Many of the effects that produce monogamy in voles are triggered not just by oxytocin but by the right balance of oxytocin and vasopressin. In all of this, there is not a straightforward, dose-dependent response to oxytocin, no rule that says more oxytocin yields more warm and fuzzy behavior. Rather, these adaptive social traits emerge from a complex dance between the two neuropeptides—at least these two—and then play into a cascade of hormones. And all is gender-dependent.

But a second element of this discussion looms even larger. Oxytocin and vasopressin are molecules that carry a signal of sorts, and there need to be receptors in the brain specific to each molecule. The number and efficacy of these receptors have much to do with how the brain reads and accomplishes the effects called for in the cascade of these molecules and all the other neuropeptides that the body uses to regulate the mind. Indeed, the research has targeted these very receptors from the beginning. For instance, researchers, as we said, were able to make the normally inattentive and philandering male meadow voles behave like the monogamous and responsible prairie voles. But they did so not by amping up oxytocin levels but by genetically engineering vole brains for better receptors. Oxytocin is a universal chemical in vertebrate life, but the differences among the various species' behaviors are due in part to variations in receptors, not levels of oxytocin. This also explains why the trait of monogamy is not a neat, linear progression through evolutionary family trees, but rather pops up here and there. Genes that build the receptors kick in and out, like toggle switches.

Researchers also believe that the variability in receptors helps explain differences within species, why one individual is more touchy-feely than another. This is not the sole explanation. As we have seen, exercise or encountering the right mate triggers spikes in oxytocin, but genes play a role as well. Genes control, at least in part, the number of receptors, and that very idea is why Carter bristles at the current simplistic line of research that says all we need to do is spritz a bit of oxytocin up one's nose to provoke a lifetime of sweetness and light. Her caution is based on some hard research and some personal experience.

A postdoc working with Carter, Karen Bales recently completed work in voles meant to mimic the effect of giving autistic children a few squirts of oxytocin while they were young—and while the animals were young, the treatment worked as expected, making for warmer and fuzzier adolescent prairie voles. But as they aged, their behavior began to deviate from the norms of polite prairie vole society. That is, these same males had a hard time partnering up. Those early doses made them less, not more, social as adults.

Carter told us she thinks those early doses of oxytocin are, in effect, "downregulating"—that is, desensitizing—the normal receptors of those young voles. As they age, then, the receptors are less able to read normal levels of oxytocin.

And this is where her line of logic becomes at once deeply personal and near universal. Despite being the world's go-to expert on oxytocin, Carter was treated pretty much like any other delivering mother in a hospital in Germany a generation ago. Back then, she told us, it was relatively rare for doctors to inject mothers in labor with the synthetic form of oxytocin, Pitocin—it happened in maybe 10 percent of deliveries. But she was injected.

"This concerns me a great deal, and it concerned me right from the start," she said. "As a scientist, I wanted to know what I did to my baby by letting the doctor give me that, but I really didn't have a choice."

True, the doctors did not give the drug to the baby, but now we know that this same molecule shows up in the brain seconds after a mere mist of it is in the air, and a baby in utero is far more intimately connected to the source. Carter must think about this now, knowing as she does the results that showed up in those prairie voles only when they became adults. A very recent paper correlates an increase in the incidence of autism with receiving Pitocin during delivery. Carter says that Pitocin is routinely administered to delivering mothers in, she estimates, 90 percent of cases, although there are some signs that this practice is waning.

At the same time, the current spate of research has turned up some other drawbacks to this simplistic, medical-model approach to oxytocin and vasopressin—but these are as intriguing as they are cautionary. These findings open a window to some sobering realizations about evolution itself and our ability to comprehend its wisdom. They make us confront violence.

What one tends to remember and report from those early prairie vole experiments is that the neuropeptides in question provoked monogamy, bonding, and solid parenting—true enough. But Carter says it was also true from the beginning that once the adolescent male crossed the line of puberty in a chemical rush, he ceased to be a meek little field mouse. "He becomes a lethal weapon," she said. "He fights off any and all intruders and will fight to the death at the same time he is the nurturing father and devoted mate."

In its summary of research on oxytocin, *Science* magazine reported on a study in Amsterdam headed by Cartsen De Dreu that used a nasal dose of oxytocin and assessed the effects with a standard game that subjects played for money:

Compared with men who got a saline spray, those who sniffed oxytocin behaved more altruistically to members of their own team—but at the same time, they were more likely to preemptively punish competitors....In a 2011 study in the Proceedings of the National Academy of Sciences, De Dreu's team found that oxytocin increased favoritism toward subjects' own ethnic group (native Dutch men) on a series of tasks and thought experiments done on a computer, and in some situations the treated men exhibited more prejudice against other groups (Germans and Middle Easterners, in this case).

This is a double-edged sword.

One goal of oxytocin research has been to promote desirable characteristics like trust, empathy, and loyalty, traits in short supply among us today. Yet we may want to place our assessment of "desirable" in context with a question that Carter put to us: if science could indeed deliver a pill that would make you a paragon of these very traits, would you take it?

And you need not think long to answer in the negative. That distrust of outsiders often leads to violence against those same people, and in evolutionary terms, violence is not necessarily a problem. Violence is useful and therefore adaptive; we need it to survive and always have. Even today, in situations where violence seems to be counteradaptive, it persists because in so many other situations it was critical to survival.

We did not get our first hint of this conclusion from biochemistry or even from evolutionary history. John Ratey has a long history of treating some exceedingly violent people, and a clear theme emerged in his practice, especially in dealing with domestic violence. The blowup and the violence in those situations (and this is not a trivial matter at all; by far, domestic violence is our most widespread form of violence in modern society) often come at a critical and common point: when the victim, the female, takes steps to leave an abusive partner. That threat triggers an irrational rage that quickly explodes—and it took time to see it, but it became clear to John that this explosion was defensive. The partner's threat to leave was a threat to the home, and the violence—no matter how irrational or misplaced—was a defense of the home.

We are not arguing that this sort of violence is justified or even adaptive. It is, in fact, a failure of the brain's coping mechanisms when faced with threat. The executive function of the brain in the frontal cortex gets hijacked in these situations, and violence ensues. It is irrational and pathological—but the wiring for it, the tendency, was put in place by evolution as an adaption. It is precisely the same impulse that sorts us into tribes, that causes us to feel best when in the circle of like-minded people we were born into and feel ill at ease when we are among others, maybe Ju/wasi, Masai, Apache, and Sarmatian once, now maybe Christians or Muslims, Republicans or Democrats, immigrants, operagoers, gardeners, bluegrass musicians, or the folks we know at the CrossFit gym. Distrust of outsiders is the flip side of the social bonding that allows us to trust those closest to us.

THE CORE HUMAN TRAIT

We deliberately entered this broader discussion of tribalism and violence through oxytocin because childbirth, nurturing, and

212 • GO WILD

bonding lie at the center of the human experience. Early in this book, we outlined the broad markers of human evolution and introduced this key point. Now it is time to revisit it in this new context.

We need only consider the cartoon image of cavemen in modern imagination to begin to understand our long-blinkered perception of the nature of our ancestors: in the cartoons, the caveman always carries a club. This is nothing more than an extension of the Hobbesian notion of nastiness, meanness, brutishness, et cetera, yet the notion is not limited to cartoons. Throughout paleoanthropology, there has been a persistent strain of imagining our species' development as governed by violence. Much of this has been rooted in the study of bones, skeletal remains that show signs of breaks and stabs and beatings, and so people reading these bones from time to time interpreted this as a sign of constant warfare.

At the same time, our closest living relatives—even the comparably peaceful bonobo, but especially chimpanzees—show plenty of ability when it comes to violence, even warfare, and so this, too, is part of the state of nature. Further, we have seen it emerge in the inquiries of people like Carrier, who began by looking at our body's adaptation for running but wound up concluding that we are equally adapted for and well suited to punching and throwing spears. Truly, violence is in our bones and muscle. This conclusion will not go away, evident also in the headlines of the day, the confirmation of hatred and carnage in our times and in all times. Indeed, the evolutionary psychologist Steven Pinker has argued that we in fact live in relatively peaceful times, and that the record shows the past has been characterized by stunning degrees of aggression toward one another far worse than today. He argues that a decline in violence is a benefit of civilization and that slowly humanity is learning to put this aside. We can only hope. Yet there are some lessons from evolution that may help us think about this most vexing of human dilemmas.

Pinker's argument is data-based, and he argues that it holds through all of human history—yet there is good reason to make the distinction that we have throughout this book: that the best evidence for our violent past comes from the past ten thousand years, a time when territory and ownership of land became vital, when farms supported cities, when monarchs could raise armies, and when we developed the tools for mass warfare. Much of the case that hunter-gatherers spent a great deal of time and energy killing one another is circumstantial at best. For instance, one analysis of the bumps and breaks on ancient skeletons—evidence earlier interpreted as resulting from warfare—got another look from researchers who found a close modern analogue to skeletons in this condition, and these were not the skeletons of warriors. The closest match to injuries like these in modern times were in rodeo cowboys, people who mix it up with big unruly animals for sport.

Some distinctions need to be drawn, and saying that primitive life was rough-and-tumble is not the same as saying it was violent.

It may help to be a bit more precise in our definitions. First, we would argue that hunting is not violence. It is killing, true enough. There will be blood. But the brain of the hunter is in a very different mode than the brain of a murderer or warrior. This is pretty clear-cut and demonstrable in measurable phenomena like brain waves. The hunter generally faces no threat that triggers a response of terror or aggression. Just the opposite, as we have seen on so many levels. The hunter is engaged, even empathetic. Indeed, through every bit of knowledge we have of hunting peoples—from the cave paintings in southern France to the rituals of plains bison hunters—comes evidence that these people regarded their prey with respect and awe.

Beyond, there seems to be a good case for separating out defensive violence against predators. Beating off lions and bears is not what we think about today when we discuss violence, yet fighting off predators probably was the form of fighting we knew best in evolutionary times. The threat of predation shaped us, and it had to, particularly the threat to our helpless infants. When we speak of violence as adaptive in evolutionary terms, this is the best example. This is why aggression is the flip side of the bonding powers of oxytocin; it is adaptive not only to cooperate and bond with our fellows but to protect and defend.

Yet none of this gets at aggression against other humans, and it should. Why does aggression persist beyond reasons for it? Why are we so riven with senseless killing and warfare? Is this simply who we are, as Pinker argues, and does this require the cultural evolution of civilization to gradually wear it away, wall it off to a silent corner of our gene pool?

Part of our thinking about human evolution has missed a great deal because we see what we want to see, and the caveman with the club is something of an icon in this regard. We are indeed fascinated by broken bones, spear points, and stacks of mutilated skeletons, yet much has been gained in reexamining the evidence from a different perspective. Put another way, the history of trying to understand human evolution has been beset with all sorts of debates about what defined us, what came first, and what is most important. Big brain? Opposable thumbs and use of tools? Fire? Fishing? In all of this there is an obvious bias toward things men do.

Yet one of the more thoughtful and interesting students of human evolution, the anthropologist Sarah Blaffer Hrdy, has told us much by reexamining the evidence in light of the things women do. In terms of evolution, her approach represents far more than correcting a gender bias. In evolutionary terms, the success of a species is completely dependent on reproduction—whether it goes on, and whether it fields a set of genes for the next generation. As we have said, *Homo sapiens* are unique in all the animal world, completely without precedent in one regard. No other species must spend as much time and energy rearing and protecting infants as we do. To Hrdy, this is the defining fact of our existence, and the term she uses is "cooperative breeding." That is, we come together as a species to raise children: "What I want to stress here, however, is that cooperative breeding was the *preexisting condition* [emphasis hers] that permitted the evolution of these traits in the hominin line. Creatures may not need big brains to evolve cooperative breeding, but hominins needed shared care and provisioning to evolve big brains. Cooperative breeding had to come first."

She is saying our cooperation and ability to bond to one another is primal, foundational, the bedrock. In her book *Mothers and Others,* she hits on the essence of this idea: "Brains require care more than caring requires brains."

Still, the persistence of violence seems to contradict the importance of bonding, but then humans are nothing if not contradictions. And this contradiction teases out an even more basic issue of evolution—one that today's evolutionary biologists debate at great length, but which has in recent years produced all sorts of insights into the forces that drive us. Much of evolutionary thought has rested on discussions of individual fitness, with an individual being a discrete unit of genes, and therefore the only unit on which evolution can act. Yet as studies of social animals (ants, termites, prairie voles, and humans) came to the fore, it occurred to thinkers that there was such a thing as group fitness. That is, the degree to which we were able to successfully cooperate and cohere as groups yielded clear advantages to our survival. This raised the idea of group rather than individual selection, a notion still hotly debated. And whether we know it or not, it is still hotly debated every day and every second in each of our brains. That's because it is sometimes to our advantage to do what is good for us as individuals and other times to do what is best for the group—selfish behavior versus altruistic behavior. Both confer advantages in evolutionary terms, and we are wired to heed both sets of messages.

It's best at this point to return to the evolutionary biologist E. O. Wilson: "The human condition is an endemic turmoil rooted in the evolution processes that created us. The worst in our nature coexists with the best, and so it will ever be. To scrub it out, if such were possible, would make us less than human."

9

Central Nerves

How the Body Wires Together Health and Happiness

Let's go back to the town house near Chapel Hill, North Carolina. Sue Carter's husband, an intense-looking fellow, had met us at the door, introduced himself in a businesslike way, and retreated so we could talk with Carter. Later, there was a break in our conversation, and he was rummaging around in the kitchen, opening drawer after drawer, searching for the tamper for his espresso machine, a clear case of partner-based misplacement of crucial accessories.

"Sue puts things away, and I look for things," he announces without preamble. "I've decided it's all about the other person thinking you know exactly what they are doing. The problem is the interpretation of intent and whether the feedback from it modifies behavior."

It's not apparent that an espresso tamper merits this depth of analysis, but then this guy is Stephen Porges. His career has been nothing so much as tracing a vital thread, a literal twisting, winding cord that can tie together the ideas we have been tracking in these pages. Carter studies social bonding chemistry and oxyto-cin. Porges studies the neural structure of social bonding, especially the vagus nerve. Think of it as Carter knowing the software and Porges specializing in the hardware. But this nerve is also where all the topics we've been thinking about seem to converge, in signals along the vagus and the central nervous system, in which it is a key player. Remember that when we considered the sweep of evolution and its intention for our well-being, it brought us ultimately to social bonding; the whole business—the brain, exercise, eating, minding, and sleeping—traced in the end to our need to deal with one another, to empathy and altruism. More than any of our other signature traits, these two require the most brain power and allow us to be who we are, the most social of social animals. These are the capstones. And when we parse that out, especially when considering the evolutionary context—our deep history as pieces of meat for predators—then all of this must have something to do with stress, fear, terror, and dealing with these matters in order to survive.

Elizabeth Marshall Thomas, the writer who spent her formative years with African hunter-gatherers, writes a great deal about lions in her account of the San people of the Kalahari. The San people she knew did indeed face lions as predators, as all people have for almost all of time. Yet these people seemed to have a finely wrought and intricate relationship with lions, the animals that owned the night. "Among the people we knew, only lions generated profound respect," she wrote.

"Respect." Not "terror," but "respect."

Thomas witnessed a number of confrontations between lions and the San people and describes nowhere any reaction that looks the slightest bit like panic. No one ran from lions. No one froze in fear. No one, certainly, engaged in fight. So here it is, the fundamental, raw, tooth-and-bone confrontation with the barest facts of biology, and yet there's no evidence whatsoever of resorting to the basic biological mechanisms for terror: fight, flight, or freeze. Instead, there is respect.

But there is more in the specifics of what is really going on. Far from fleeing a lion, San people had a "protocol" (Thomas's word)—and it involved walking. Walking calmly, unhurriedly, and not directly, as fleeing prey might, but obliquely at an angle, away from the lion. At the same time, they spoke to the lion, in well-modulated tones of respect, addressing it as "old lion."

Richard Manning has had a direct and similar personal experience with a grizzly bear in the wild and observed exactly the same protocol, accepted by bear biologists as the way to deal with these big predators. The protocol is ancient and endures and has much to say about meeting not just predators but the challenges of modern life. Porges thinks he can trace the development of that protocol in the body's most ancient and tortuous nerve, the vagus nerve—it gets its very name from the same word as "vagabond," a wanderer, a traveler, a time traveler.

THE ANCIENT NERVE

Porges is a rare bird among scientists, a guy who has spawned his very own theory of human behavior, an idea that has acolytes and practitioners and real-world, on-the-ground applications. For instance, at the Center for Discovery in New York, we met a young, bright guy from MIT, Matthew Goodwin, who had used Porges's ideas to incorporate the same sort of telemetry that lurks in the guts of an iPhone to track and predict disruptive out-breaks in autistic people. This is the sort of application that started Porges thinking about all of this decades ago — the idea of measurable, readable physical manifestations of our state of mind, a literal pulse of our psychological well-being.

The vagus nerve is the only one that attaches to the most primitive, lower part of our brain, and from there it winds the unique and circuitous course that earns it its name. Unlike most other nerves in the body, it wanders, not straight from eyeball to brain like the optic nerve but downward along the neck and then branching and twisting through the core of our body, our guts, our gonads, our viscera, and if you hear in this the word "visceral" you are hearing right. But then, oddly, parts of it twist back up through the throat to take in larynx, ears, facial mus-cles. Why this odd assortment of disparate organs and functions? What does our heart — just a pump, really — have to do with the crinkle in the corners of our eyes?

This tortuous path, starting as it does in the most primitive part of our brain, is first an evolutionary trail, and it clearly marks the vagus as ancient. It makes its straight march to the chest and heartbeat but also back upward to innervate structures that had their origins in the gills of our very distant ancestors. It is an integral part of a network known as the autonomic nervous system, which regulates automatic responses in our organs — but not only automatic responses. Among the system's key tasks is regulation of our body's response to threat, terror, and lions, the center of control for fight, flight, or freeze.

When presented with a threat, each of these strategies requires regulation throughout the territory covered by the vagus nerve and the rest of the autonomic nervous system. For instance, heart rate and respiration increase, both effects that supply extra energy for fight or flight. The digestive system shuts down to save energy. Same with the gonads. Same with immune response. Facial muscles contract and contort to the fierce presentation of rage. The larynx tightens to pitch urgent vocalizations. This is your body at DEFCON 1. And then the threat passes, and the vagus nerve reverses all of this. The whole cycle, arousal and relaxation, is an oscillation that is adaptive and serves as the successful response to danger.

In all of this, the shutdown sometimes gets taken for granted, but it is not a given. The terror response doesn't just stop on its own; it requires a whole separate set of signals to shut it down. Over time, people who are repeatedly abused or terrorized, especially as children, lose the ability to return to normal, almost as if a switch got stuck. They literally live in terror. Further, tracing the course of the autonomic nervous system shows quickly why so many issues deemed psychological play out in the body: digestive issues, impotence, poor immune response, high blood pressure, elevated heart rate, tense faces.

A curiosity about the physical manifestations of a psychological state is what brought Porges to the vagus nerve in the first place. What kept him there was the realization that the vagus nerve runs both ways. It is mostly a control nerve, signaling organs to relax, but it also sends information back up to the brain on the state of the organs.

Begin, though, by understanding that social engagement, the ability to deal with another of our species on the basis of trust and understanding, is, in terms of all animals, truly bizarre behavior. Almost no other species can do it as well as we do, and those that can, like dogs, tend to hang around with us. Porges says the reason this is so in evolutionary terms is that very few species have the ability to apply the vagal brake. The ability to calmly speak with one's spouse as to the whereabouts of the espresso tamper means asking the autonomic nervous system to perform two contradictory goals at the same time—and the key to that, says Porges, is the vagal brake. The vagus nerve links up all the tools we need to respond to an existential threat, and so the vagal brake is a signal sent through the system for everything to stand down and engage—at ease.

And it turns out there is a simple measure of this. It can be read in the tension or lack of tension in facial muscles, heard in voice timbre and edge, and counted in rate of respiration. But at the heart of the matter is the heart itself and a subtle little signal called the respiratory sinus arrhythmia. When the vagal brake is applied, it calms the heart as it does everything else, and the unequal pressures of breathing (the increase with inhalation and decrease with exhalation) actually syncopate the heartbeat with a little asymmetry in rhythm, a slight difference between contraction and expansion. This is a respiratory arrhythmia and the syncopation can be read on a graph, plain as day. Further, says Porges, there is such a thing as vagal tone, completely analogous to muscle tone—and the tone shows how clear and distinct a given individual's ability to apply the brake is. That tone can be read in the amplitude of the arrhythmia. People who are comfortable engaging other people have strong vagal tone.

For openers, this realization revitalizes a whole collection of metaphors in our language and most others by suggesting that they are more than metaphors. A strict rationalist's reading of statements like "I know it in my heart" or "My heart is not in this" sees them as a cover for mushy thinking. In strict, reductionist, mechanistic thinking, the heart is just a pump, not so different from the circulating pump in the boiler in the basement. (Likewise, science has begun talking about a "second brain" in your body: the enteric nervous system. We have long known that the digestive system has a robust set of nerves of its own, but research is finding out that this system does far more than regulate digestion. It is a full complement of neurotransmitters and, in fact, seems to play a key role in regulating your sense of well-being, both physical and mental. It plays a role in your decision process, hence "second brain." Now metaphors like "gut instinct" get some real-world traction.)

Yet it now seems as if there was an instinctive understanding in the evolution of our language that recognized what we can now measure in graphs and blips and charts: that the heart and gut are deeply engaged in our emotional lives. But this might seem a bit much on the evidence we've delivered so far. It's cool that the heartbeat gives us a measure, but so what? It's only a slightly more sophisticated measure than, say, rate of respiration, galvanic skin response, or a twitch in our facial muscles that any dog can read.

To which Porges replies, no, no. The vagal brake can be driven by breath, a clear connection readable as blips on a chart. You are in control of your breath, to some degree. Thus, this is not simply a point for measuring or sensing arousal; it is a point for controlling arousal and, downstream, the health problems that stem from lack of control.

We have long had intriguing clues as to how our body might participate in psychological health. For instance, it is a no-brainer that if you feel better, you are more likely to smile. But people studying depression figured out long ago that if you force yourself to smile, the specific spots in the brain that register depression suddenly say your depression is better. Nothing else changed in your life, so why should this be? Through the years, neuroscience has produced a refinement of this intriguing little bit of information. It turns out that a halfway, forced smile won't do the trick because it won't light up the neurons of increased happiness in your brain. But if that forced smile goes so far as to engage the little muscles in the corners of your eyes—that is, if you do what socially adept people understand instinctively—these neurons do indeed light up. And the muscles at the corners of your eyes are within the reach of the vagus nerve.

Yet where this idea really hits home is with the breath, the one response over which we have control and which, in turn, exerts control through the alarm system that is the autonomic nervous system. Porges says he realized a long time ago—because he is a musician, specifically a horn player—that the act of controlling the breath to control the rhythm of music and at the same time engaging the brain to execute the mechanics of music works like a mental therapy. To his mind, it has all the elements of pranayama yoga, a form of yoga that stresses breath control.

Breath control is common in most of yoga but also in meditation, and even in modern-day "evidence-based practices" like cognitive behavioral therapy. Relax. Take a deep breath. This act of controlling the breath has a parallel brain response of calming our instincts for fear and danger. It's easy enough to see this in deliberate practices like yoga, but the same idea applies in many more time-honored practices: choral singing, Gregorian chants, even social music like bluegrass or blues derived from the chants and work songs that African slaves developed to help them tolerate oppression.

There is, in fact, a musical thread throughout this idea.

There is a bias in the system to detect what Porges calls prosody, the rhythm and lilt we associate with music, singing, poetry, and chants. It is the form that becomes immediately apparent in our voices when we talk to animals or babies and is the language of our foundational relationships with our mothers. Prosody is the form of speech the San people used to engage lions.

All of this begins to explain a curious finding among the bones and ruins of our ancestors, such as flutes carved from the leg bones of cranes. Recall that music or evidence of music appeared fifty thousand years ago in that sudden flourish of evidence of cultural evolution that defined humans as humans—and ever since, music has loomed as a cultural universal. All known cultures and peoples make music. Yet all of this also suggests that we lose something when the crane's leg bone gets replaced by an iPod. We lose the benefits of sitting in a circle of fellow humans and driving the breath and beat that drives the music.

The psychiatrist and neuroscientist Iain McGilchrist argues that music predated language in human development, simply because it was more important, more necessary, and already developed by evolution in other animals like birds and whales. Language merely allowed communication. Music and components of music like lilt and prosody facilitated engagement, even with other animals, even with predators. It engaged the breath in its making.

CONNECTIONS TO PHYSICAL WELL-BEING

The vagus linkage suggests that these sorts of activities might well extend beyond emotional well-being simply because so many of the physical maladies of modern times play out in the territory of the vagus nerve and the enteric nervous system. Your yoga practice or your choral group may well have some leverage on your irritable bowel syndrome or the persistent pain in your neck for no apparent reason, because both of these are wired to the signal path of breath.

But what of exercise—pumping lungs and heart in exertion? Porges says it depends. Done wrong, exercise can drive the emotional response in the wrong direction because it relies on arousal—the physical arousal that is the opposite of relaxation. But this is not the contradiction it seems to be. In much of the animal world, the choice is either fully aroused or fully shut down, but the sophisticated autonomic nervous system of humans allows us to accomplish both at once. The most profound statement of our ability to deal with contradiction is sexual congress, the state that demands arousal in the most basic and heart-thumping sense, and at the same time requires maximal emotional openness and engagement—that is, trust. The standout ability of a well-adjusted human is to handle both arousal and engagement at once in this and all other forms of social intercourse.

Which turns out, in Porges's view, to be terribly relevant to that workout of yours at the gym. Simply plunking yourself on a treadmill or stationary bicycle, armoring with earbuds to shut out auditory signals from the real world, and then watching cable news loop the litany of the day's lurid images—he argues that this speaks straight to the reptilian reaches of the nerves. Remember, you are running, as in "flee." Running is a setup for working the grooves of panic. The alternative, though, is group activity, group play and exercise, the very sort of activity that humans seem to have preferred through the ages. Done right, this does indeed involve the arousal of the flee response, but also the social engagement of teammates and competitors and the rich sensory messages from nature and the outdoors. Now both arousal and engagement are activated, meaning your heart, body, and mind are fully involved in the most elaborate of social exercises. All of this puts a new layer of foundation beneath developments like Eva Selhub's and Matt O'Toole's enthusiasm for the CrossFit gym. Even more deeply, it helps us see further significance in ancient activities such as persistence hunting, always done in groups with sublime levels of engagement and communication among members. Persistence hunting also required an almost instinctive level of understanding and predicting the movements of the animal being tracked, a skill that observers recorded as based in empathy.

TRAUMA

One of the best windows into the relevance of all of this frames a view most of us would prefer to avoid, filled as it is with nightmarish visions. Because while the vagus nerve is central to our trust and social connection, it is also central to terror, and too many of us live at the reptilian level of this response.

The guy generally credited with having done more thinking about this than anyone else is trauma researcher Bessel van der Kolk. Porges talked much about trauma during our interview and at least part of the credit for that, he acknowledges, goes to his association with van der Kolk.

Van der Kolk grew up in the Netherlands, but as a young

man he came to Boston and trained as a psychiatrist and then became involved in treating veterans of the Vietnam War who were plagued with psychological difficulties as a result of their experiences. At that time, there was a vague notion of the source of those troubles, labeled in earlier wars as "shell shock" or "battle fatigue." But as a result of work during the Vietnam era, psychiatry gave this problem a formal diagnosis of post-traumatic stress disorder, or PTSD, a diagnosis that van der Kolk helped formulate.

Shortly thereafter, though, he became interested in the problem as it plagued children, and he has founded a national network sanctioned by Congress to research what he calls "developmental trauma." The difference between the problem in children and in adults is critical and serves as the main finding of the whole area of research. Child abuse occurs while a helpless brain is still physically forming, and so it locks in patterns of neural response largely through the mechanisms of fight, flight, or freeze. This means that the effects of childhood traumatic events linger, in fact dominate, well into adulthood, and in some surprising ways that speaks directly to what ails us.

The pivot point in this thinking was a landmark study taken on by the Centers for Disease Control and Prevention. It looked at seventeen thousand middle-class employed adults in California and assessed their history of childhood abuse against the primary causes of premature death in the United Sates, like heart disease, diabetes, stroke, and liver disease — our nation's most expensive public health problems. The results are head-turning. The researchers found, first, that there is a surprising amount of abuse in most people's lives — physical, mental, and sexual abuse as well as the experience of growing up with violent or alcoholic parents. More important, though, the researchers found that not only did abuse serve to predict poor health later in life, but the amount of abuse was directly related to the severity of the later health problems; it was, in the language of epidemiology, "dose-dependent."

Some of this can be explained by the usual routes. People abused as children tended to self-medicate as adults with alcohol, drugs, and cigarettes, and those behaviors in turn sponsored some of the later health problems. But the researchers performed statistical techniques to account for this and still showed a straightforward physical response to child abuse. This may seem a strange connection, unless one realizes that the diseases in question affect organs like the heart and lungs and processes like digestion and immune response, all of which falls into the territory of the vagus nerve.

"Trauma lives in the body," van der Kolk says often, an aphorism that tracks the vagus nerve but also the path of his own career. He has been known to state bluntly that despite his training and lifetime of experience in psychiatry, what he has learned through trauma has caused him to stop practicing psychotherapy. He is openly and frankly dismissive of talk therapy, labeling it "yakking."

And so one cold, gray afternoon in Boston, we found him holed up in a modest little ground-floor office in a brick town house, where we'd come to ask him what works—what makes people better.

"Trauma is about immobilization," he says. "What works is people moving together in time, rhythmically." Through the decades of his dealing with this problem, he's gotten results by making people move.

People who have been abused, especially as children, are often simply practicing the normal and adaptive response of freezing. That's the tool that evolution gave us. The trauma response is not a mental disease or failure of the genes and neurons; rather, it is a normal response to an abnormal situation. And at the same time, we are evolved and adapted to return to normal, to begin motion again, once the danger passes. The problem, especially with children but also with warriors who suffer PTSD, is that the danger and terror happen again and again and again; they become a way of life, and over time the biochemical and neurological systems for returning to normal, for modulating, for shutting down the alarm, just lock in place instead. And the body seizes up in the bargain. Maybe not in complete paralysis, but parts of the body do freeze, terrified to move.

"Immobilization without fear, which is really what society is all about, as opposed to immobilization with fear, which is what trauma is about," was the way Porges expressed this to us.

This is where van der Kolk slides from the biological evolution that has dominated our discussion so far to the idea of cultural evolution. His reasoning is this: Humans have dealt with terror and psychic injury for as long as there have been humans, and certainly as long as there have been lions, and more certainly as long as there have been wars. So we have developed time-tested—no, deep-time-tested—methods of coping. Van der Kolk looks for these methods, and he finds them in places you might expect, all in line with his foundation tenets of moving rhythmically together, controlling breath, and feeling the vibrations of voice. He practices yoga himself and prescribes it for others. He likes the ancient Chinese practice of qigong, a form of ritualized movement. Meditation, certainly. Many forms of dance, and chanting. He pays particular attention to theater, citing examples such as successful projects in troubled high schools, where students—many of them the victims of violence—write, rehearse, and stage musical theater as a means of recovering from the damage. One such project, called Shakespeare in the Courts and headed by the actor Tina Packer, specializes in Shakespearean theater, summoning as it does the primal cadence and earthiness of Anglo-Saxon words like "murder," "father," and "blood" to tap and relate emotional content in public.

There's nothing new about any of this. Van der Kolk points to the roots of Western theater in Greek tragedy, performances of which were filled with more public venting of emotion than modern theater is today. He believes that these rituals developed in what were then unarguably violent societies for many of the same reasons this sort of thing works in a modern context. The elements align nicely with what we are learning about emotional trauma and the intricacies of our visceral nervous system. Breath control, rhythm, whole-body movement, narrative, social ties and cues—all of these are physical impulses that travel at the literal core of our being.

Besides, he says, "people cannot rhythmically move together without beginning to giggle." Laughter trumps trauma.

BEYOND STRESS

There is a word, an overused, worn-out, imprecise, deflated word, that comes up when we talk about danger and challenge. "Stress? We shouldn't use the word," says Porges. "I think it's a bad word."

And now we've gone and done it, opened a can of worms that is in fact going to cause us to backtrack on another word, one that has served us well in our discussion so far. But once you deflate the idea of stress, then you also begin to undermine the notion of homeostasis, which is precisely what we need to do now. Homeostasis? Old hat. Last week's news. Think, instead, allostasis.

The fact that some enterprising folks in the tech world began marketing a new sort of household thermostat makes this distinction easy to analogize. Homeostasis is like a thermostat — in some cases, it behaves exactly like one. Exert yourself on a hot day and your body temperature rises above its set point of 98.6; you begin to sweat so that evaporation and cooling return you to your set point. This is homeostasis, the body's mechanism for maintaining stability at set points, such as heart rate, respiration, blood pressure, hunger, thirst, and on and on. And it's just like the sort of thermostat that hangs on the wall. Set a temperature and a furnace or an air conditioner kicks in appropriately to maintain it. Or at least that's how it worked for a hundred or so years.

But the newer, high-tech thermostats actually remember changes you make in room temperature according to conditions, not through a simple memory and program. They actually learn, remember, and predict your behavior. So they know when you get up on a cold day, and they turn up the heat in advance, just as you would do.

This, argues the new thinking, is more in line with how your body works, only your body is even more sophisticated — because unlike the thermostat on your wall, humans have big brains. The neuroscientist Peter Sterling laid out the difference in the introduction to a key paper on the topic, offering the beginnings of an idea that is providing some needed traction for our thinking:

The premise of the standard regulatory model, "homeostasis," is flawed: the goal of regulation is *not* to preserve constancy of the internal milieu. Rather, it is to continually *adjust* the milieu to promote survival and reproduction. Regulatory mechanisms need to be efficient, but homeostasis (error-correction by feedback) is inherently *inefficient*. Thus, although feedbacks are certainly ubiquitous, they could not possibly serve as the primary regulatory mechanism.

A newer model, "allostasis," proposes that efficient regulation requires *anticipating* needs and preparing to satisfy them *before* they arise.

Put another way, homeostasis can deliver only stability, and in life, stability is literally a dead-end strategy. The only stable condition of a biological organism is dead. Your body's systems must allow for growth, which means more than simply adjusting for existing conditions. Your vital systems must roll with the punches today and build capacity to absorb future punches.

We have already seen the fundamental design feature of this at work, and it goes beyond the example of the high-tech thermostat. A thermostat controls one system in your home, but your body is made up of a series of interlocking systems: circulation, digestion, immune, nervous, endocrine, and so forth. Sterling points out what any designer of an efficient car already knows. If each of those systems needed its own energy reserves and capacity to meet all needs at all times independently, the whole system would be inherently overdesigned and inefficient. Better, then, to allow energy borrowing between the systems, just as we have seen. Fight, flight, or freeze shuts down the digestive and immune systems simply to allow the muscles to use that energy instead.

Yet that same principle explains exactly why it makes no sense to treat a particular malfunction or disease by considering only one system. The overload that is producing the problem may be in another part of the body altogether, which is why "psychological" problems like PTSD show up as digestive issues and can be treated in the body. Or why, for that matter, Carol Worthman's contention that we pay for sleep deprivation in the currency of stress is true. The body is making adjustments throughout the system to meet immediate needs, and all of this is checked and balanced by the brain. At the same time, though, this system is looking to the future, both short-term, in seasonal cycles, and long-term, in changes in the conditions of life.

One example of a short-term systemic change comes as days lengthen in the spring. At this time of year, we react to increasing sunlight by producing skin pigment that protects us from increasing sunlight later in the year. Another example is that most mammals store fat as winter approaches.

But long-term regulation seems even more critical in light of the issues that have concerned us throughout this book, and we have already seen examples of just how long-term we might mean by this. Remember the research that concluded that the best predictor of obesity in children was low birth weight. The fetus senses the conditions that produce low birth weight in utero as a predictor of a lifetime of scarce resources, and so his body adjusts by becoming good at storing fat. This is not a disease or a malfunction, really, but an adaptation. But remember, too, that an important predictor of an infant's low birth weight is his mother's low birth weight, meaning the body is setting in those adaptive processes across generations.

We always assume that the method for transmitting traits across generations is genetic. For a long time, science has made much of genetic predisposition, and certainly genes play a role in governing our lives. But it is also true that much was made of genes because at the time we happened to know a lot about genes; that is, we were looking for the car keys where the light was best. In recent years, though, a whole new field has exploded on the scene: epigenetics, which is the study of gene regulation, how it is influenced by environment, and how it is inherited across generations. Much will be illuminated by this line of inquiry, but it has already pointed to one key mechanism, and, in fact, we have already seen it in action in a couple of areas we have talked about.

Remember Sue Carter's worries about oxytocin doses to infants based on the research that showed how young voles given nasal doses of oxytocin had weird relationships as adults? Her explanation was a "downregulation" of receptors. That is, the voles' bodies still produced the oxytocin, but the brain had adjusted to the excess by turning down the sensitivity of special cells that detect the signals—thus, downregulation. Sterling identifies this as a key mechanism in allostasis: the body's ability to adjust to variations in the environment, a recalibration of its instruments.

His paper on this says: "Thus, when blood glucose is persistently elevated and triggers persistent secretion of insulin, insulin receptors eventually anticipate high insulin and down-regulate. The system learns that blood glucose is *supposed* to be high." This is the smoking gun for insulin resistance, the very issue that lies at the heart of our worst health problems, like obesity, diabetes, and heart disease. It is our bodies' collective response to a long-term change in the conditions of life wrought by industrial agriculture and processed food.

Yet wrapped in this sort of adaptation for change is the mechanism for growth, and it, too, is rooted in what we might call stress. This is the process at work in every long run uphill or in every set of bench presses that reaches for a new personal record. We build muscles by tearing them down, stressing them beyond their limits. The body reads this as a need for more muscle to meet these new conditions of your life, and so the body builds it. And this works the same way in the brain: brain-building chemicals build new cells and make existing cells stronger.

Yet Sterling's paper refines this line of thought by pointing out that the brain is not simply executing all of these controls on autopilot, but is in fact engaging our consciousness and sense of well-being in the entire process. The brain is wired with what he labels a set of carrots and sticks that move each of us to adapt and respond along with the rest of the body. Pain is a part of this—surely a big stick—but more intriguing is the degree to which all of these circuits for adaptation are tied directly to our brain's dopamine circuits, the pleasure circuits and the brain's reward system. Sterling makes the same argument we heard from Robert Sapolsky when we talked about meditation. That is, we get the greatest pleasure not out of a predictable reward but out of an unexpected one. We take pleasure in challenge and get more mindful and focused at the same time by dopamine, which is the carrot pulling us along to overcome the challenges of survival, short- and long-term.

The flip side of this is anxiety, the stick that pushes us in elemental fears, the most common and elemental fear being, at least in evolutionary times, concern over where your next meal is coming from. The relief arrives in a squirt of dopamine that is the result of answering that concern every day. Sterling writes this: "*Sensitivity* to dopamine also declines because dopamine receptors, anticipating high levels, have down-regulated. This may explain Goethe's famous remark, '*Nothing is harder to bear than a succession of fair days.*'"

Yet in engineering a society that is nothing so much as a succession of fair days, we have removed the dopamine reward, and so we go mindlessly looking for ways to replace it. Some of us climb mountains or ride roller coasters. More commonly, though, the void gets filled with a suite of addictions, especially to drugs and alcohol, which play to the dopamine circuits, now governed by downregulated receptors that leave us asking for more.

All of this suggests that the strategy for coping is not removing stress, or what we call stress, from our lives. Rather, as we have argued throughout, the real problem, the killer, is the chronic, unrelenting, unremitting series of regular events that wears us down. You can skip a night's sleep now and again. It may, in fact, even be good for you to do so. But not day after day. You can tolerate and even thrive on astounding variety and variability in your diet, even enjoying an occasional slice of chocolate cake, but the daily, unrelenting dose of Big Gulp Cokes will kill you. Every runner knows you build strength on rest days. Dealing with a lion every now and again makes you better at dealing with lions. Allowing your life to surmount occasional challenges is inoculation—almost literally—against future stress.

This brings us back to a central point in this book: variety. Remember, we argued from the beginning that the hallmark of the human condition is our ability to tolerate and thrive and in a wide variety of conditions—the Swiss Army knife model. So if our tolerance for variety is so great, how can we argue that modern life, with all its apparent variety—wheat, sugar, agriculture, iPads, noise, and the rest—is killing us? Much of that answer lies in deciding who each of us is.

The neuroendocrinologist Bruce S. McEwen and the researcher Linn Getz build on Sterling's idea of allostasis by using it to form a strategy of personalized medicine that involves employing specific and complex information about each individual to decide on interventions for problems. This idea has some currency in mainstream, medical-model medicine, but usually it is couched in terms of genetics. An individual's course of treatment would depend on sequencing his genome to decide his genetic predisposition to disease and its cures.

Yet McEwen and Getz argue that this ignores epigenetics and life history and that those influences are if anything more important. Specifically, they argue that there is such a thing as "orchid" children and "dandelion" children, individuals sorted by their specific tolerance for variability and challenge as shaped by the events in their lives. Dandelion children thrive anywhere; orchids are hothouse flowers. How far one goes in the direction of novel challenge and how attentive one needs to be to a safe, familiar base is a matter of where one falls on the orchid-dandelion continuum, and this is true for adults as well as children. But over time, with effort, one can move toward the dandelion end of the scale. This is growth. This is building resilience by inoculation against stress. This is re-wilding.

The idea summons an image we used to introduce this book, the common scene employed in teaching students of child development: mother and toddler alone in a room, toddler clinging to mother to draw strength and foundation and courage, and then using that base to leave mother to explore, to be challenged, and then being surprised in fear and retreating to mother for reassurance. And then, if mother is good and does her job well, toddler explores again and grows.

This is not just for toddlers. The evolutionary conditions that shaped us are that base of comfort and strength, the mother. Gather that strength and then venture forth to explore the variety and wonder of the world, the wild. And when it jolts you, pull back, rest, and grow among people you love and trust. Whether you're stressed or relaxed, well-being is not about always being safe or fed or comfortable. Rather, it is learning to walk the line between the two, to balance, to move back and forth between them with ease and grace. Well-being comes from learning to talk to the lions.

10

Personal Implications

What We Did and What You Can Do

Indeed, the sources of our happiness are complicated, rooted as they are in the complexity of our bodies, but also, as we have argued, in the complexities of the twists and turns of our individual life stories, all of which forces the conclusion that there is no single prescription for well-being. Given this, the temptation is to paraphrase our favorite advice on writing from the great journalist A. J. Liebling: The only way to live is well, and how you do that is your own damned business.

But this is a cop-out of sorts. There is a better way to deal with this matter of personal prescription: Our bodies and minds are endowed by evolution with marvelous systems tuned to attend to our happiness. Our task is to learn to listen to those systems and stay out of their way. As we argued in the beginning: if this grail of well-being is so elusive, so unattainable, then why can hunter-gatherers who have never heard of the scientific marvels that we have cited here achieve what we are after without even really trying?

Yes, living organisms are complex, but now it's time to shift gears and deliver, as we promised, some synthesis of all of this that you might use in your own life. Both authors have learned through years of public appearances that audiences will often ask a pointed question that eliminates the cop-out of not offering a prescription: "Yeah, but what do *you* do?"

There are a lot of scientific uncertainties and dueling studies that plague this issue. But the simple and necessary realization is that in all really interesting questions of science, there is no such thing as certainty. And yet there is a certainty that each of us must live a life, and each of us must make the choices that guide that process.

We—each of the authors—did not hatch and assemble the ideas that brought us to this point solely from within the confines of research, inquiry, conversation, and logic. These notions came to us like most: after years of living. This book is not an academic exercise for either of us, but rather a product of living our real and textured lives. So, each in his turn, we are now going to give you some parts of our personal stories, especially recent parts, when we used our own bodies as laboratories for exploring these ideas. The truth is, our lives changed greatly during the process of writing this book—changed for the better. And we think that our experiences might offer some guideposts for your own explorations.

JOHN RATEY

Probably like many of you reading this, my life can be described as hectic, overscheduled, too much to do with too little time. In addition to running a psychiatric practice in Cambridge, Massachusetts, I teach, lecture around the world, write books and papers—and if that isn't enough, I have a bicoastal relationship with my wife, Alicia, a television producer in Los Angeles, which sends me on planes back and forth between the coasts.

Over the years, I have certainly been guilty of getting too little sleep, grabbing a hot dog and a soda on the run, being too wired after spending hours at the computer returning email, checking the news, the latest science reports, and even the New England Patriots scores. In the city jungles of Boston and L.A., "nature" is not readily available, and certainly finding quality time to spend with my tribe, recently made bigger by the important addition of my very first grandchild, hasn't always been easy.

But change can happen. If I can incorporate the concepts laid out in this book in my own hectic life, thereby creating a healthier physical self along with a greater sense of emotional well-being, so can you. Of course, my life didn't start out in so many directions, at a frenzied and sometimes unhealthy pace. When I look back on my childhood, I see how "wild" I really was without even knowing it. I grew up in Beaver, Pennsylvania, a small town outside Pittsburgh, where we lived in a real old-style neighborhood. "Tribe" was important. Beaver was a place where everybody knew and cared for one another, with the usual crabs and discontented folks, but mainly people who were strivers of Tom Brokaw's greatest generation. Our food was natural and home-cooked. My mother always had a garden, and we delighted in the fresh summer tastes of tomatoes, onions, leaf lettuce, and carrots. Sleep was regimented, and when the day ended, there was little TV, let alone the digital life that wires us now. Rather than playing video games or texting friends, my job was to play vigorously with my close band of buddies, Fred and Joe, and we were always on the move. From almost the time we could walk, it seemed that every kid in town was playing Little League on the field or touch football on a neighbor's front lawn. We were frequently in the elements, running through the nearby woods playing cowboys and Indians, putting our architectural prowess to the test as we built forts in the backyard with giant piles of leaves, or just doing nothing as we sat on the banks of the Ohio River fishing for carp and catfish.

As I grew up, my understanding of sleep, diet, movement, nature, meditation, and the importance of connection also grew. Over the years, I've been fortunate to delve into these areas, taught by some of the most impressive academic and professional minds out there. Looking back, I now see where, even as lessons were being firmly implanted into my intellectual self, in my personal life, I frequently moved farther and farther away from my wild child days and my inherent genetic roots.

Upon moving away from Beaver and on to medical school, sleep was one of the first things to go. I was surviving on fumes, burning the candle at both ends as a medical student and resident at Massachusetts Mental Health Center. If I could have, I would have stayed awake 24-7, because this was the mecca of psychiatric training. There I met with the world famous sleep researcher Dr. Allan Hobson. The irony is, although I was sleep-deprived then, he would become a good friend, guide, and mentor. We spent our days and nights in a lab, observing animal behavior in studies of sleep onset and trying to unpack what sleep was. This was the beginning of neuroscience; sleep was a subject of great interest, and it seemed as though we would discover what it was for. But as we said in our sleep chapter, we still do not know that answer. We just know we need sleep.

I knew that eight hours was necessary for a good night's sleep, but in my whole life I had never gotten close to this regimen. I was the wellness revolutionary who was proud of how little sleep he needed and even bragged about it. I realize now how wrong this was, and today I see that the more sleep I get, the better.

The head and emotional leader of the department was Elvin Semrad. He was all about connecting with your patients and their bodies, how they felt, and how you could empathize with them. He shooed us away from constructs and reading, and instead got us to observe ourselves in the moment. We needed to be present with our patients to deeply understand how they felt, both in their body and at an unconscious level. This wasn't about a symptom checklist but about being mindful and getting them to be mindful of how and where they were in pain.

Connection is one of the most important tenets of my personal life as well. I do not work or live well alone, and so family, friends, and coworkers are a constant support. My good friend and collaborator Ned Hallowell is a champion at emphasizing the need to work at this, to create the time and rituals to connect regularly with friends. But the power of this was quite evident. We needed to ritualize it with ironclad times, or it would go away. I always created or joined groups that interested me and kept me going professionally. Bessel van der Kolk and others started a group focused on trauma, attention, and neuroscience, and we have met every second Monday of the month for more than twenty years, with frequent guest speakers on a wide variety of subjects. I have never written alone and have a new tribe formed with Dick Manning.

Along with appreciating the power of connection, I have

had a profound respect for the effect of movement on our brains and psyches. Exercise is deeply ingrained in my DNA and I feel it. From my early days in medical school, I saw the power of movement and its ability to regulate emotional well-being. In medical school, I saw an article about a hospital in Norway that was admitting depressed patients and offering our then brand-new miracle drugs (the antidepressants that effected norepinephrine) or an exercise program three times a day. The hospital claimed that each treatment had the same results. This stuck with me during my residency, when the Boston Marathon was just booming—everyone, or almost everyone, was training for the marathon, or at least running.

In the '70s we had just discovered endorphins, and everyone was talking about the endorphin rush and its power to stave off depression (simplistic causality was the rule). Then I learned that drugs that approximated the effects of chronic exercise and meditation—the beta-blockers, which act to tamp down the drive of the sympathetic nervous system and allow the parasympathetic to take over—were useful for aggression, violence, autistic disruptive behaviors, self-abuse, anxiety, social anxiety, stress-related disorders in general, and certainly attention deficit disorder. The magical effect of exercise on my own and others' attention systems led to a whole career of writing about ADHD, then to the brain itself, and finally to exercise, in my most recent book, *Spark: The Revolutionary New Science of Exercise and the Brain*. After reviewing more than a thousand papers for this book, I redoubled my efforts to exercise daily despite my overly jammed schedule. I run, use the gym frequently to provide the scaffolding for other activities, and love hiking, and a big part of most vacations is physical activity in the mountains or near the water.

With all my training and access to the greatest minds at Harvard and MIT, the interconnectedness of concepts in this book never really hit me until a chance encounter at a gym in a small town on the eastern coast of northern Michigan. It was here that I met Casey Stutzman, who would send me on a journey I never anticipated.

It was here, while on vacation with my wife, that I put the final pieces of the puzzle together. Alicia's family cottage is fairly "wild." We were surrounded by nature, with the beauty of Lake Huron at our doorstep. We relished sleeping in until we were no longer tired, and it was the perfect environment to connect with each other and disconnect from the world. The only Internet connection involved a drive to the local library.

Of course, exercise is always a must, and wherever we are in the world, Alicia and I seek out a gym or a hike. Being in Harrisville, Michigan, was no exception. It meant a forty-five-minute drive to the biggest city in the area, Alpena, a town of thirteen thousand, in what some would consider the middle of nowhere. By the oddest of coincidences, though, it is the town where Dick was raised, leading me to believe there's something special in the waters of the Great Lakes. It was at the gym connected to the regional hospital rehab center that we met an enthusiastic, cutting-edge trainer, Casey Stutzman. Always expanding his knowledge and introducing the community to the latest development, he was offering Tabata and TRX training well before our fancy Los Angeles and Boston health clubs did. Casey incorporates fun and challenge into each hour, and every year since that first we've looked forward to our week away from the madding crowd in part because it means working with him. After one very challenging class, I told him we had just signed on to write this book, and he immediately piped up about his wife Mary Beth's life-changing experience when she began a new diet—how bad she had been feeling, and how it had saved her life. He had also changed his diet and found that he had a lot more energy, focus, and joy in his life. This inspired me, and I began to both change my diet and make sure I got outside more.

Like many of my colleagues, I had been lowering my carbohydrate and trans fat intake for years, but now I approached this with new vigor and commitment. I concentrated on eliminating all grains from my diet. That meant no more pizzas, crackers, rice, or pasta. Finally, I gave up breads, which I had previously devoured. I added more vegetables and fruits to my usual fare and began to appreciate nuts as an easy, delicious, and filling snack. Also, I started to notice that the cream in my coffee led to a GI reaction, so I stopped that ritual and found that I actually enjoyed black coffee.

In about six weeks, I lost ten pounds; I was close to my weight in high school. I was never overweight but had gotten a little soft around the middle like most people my age.

Now Alicia calls me "faux paleo" because I still have Manhattans when I am in a bar or a restaurant. I'm fanatical about the diet—and it's difficult to be, given my travel schedule, but I do notice that in restaurants and even in airports things are changing a bit, with low-carb options and farm-to-table offerings becoming more prevalent.

I have to watch myself, as I can tend to drop below my high school weight; then I have to splurge on a pasta dinner or take a break from my usual diet for a day or two. I've found that I am now more "mindful" of my food and more open to new tastes and textures; I enjoy greater variety.

I want to emphasize that I am not a paleo zealot, and I am never hungry. I have seen a great change in my energy and mood, and I no longer have the midafternoon slump I used to have before I adopted this extraordinary low-carb diet. I sleep better and have more exercise stamina, and even with my hectic schedule, my energy remains. I am hooked.

At about the same time that my "re-wilding" was taking place, I joined an extraordinary group of researchers and caregivers on a massive project to investigate the effects of "smart living" on 360 adolescents with autism at the Center for Discovery in Harris, New York. There, on a hundred-acre farm in the middle of the Catskills, an amazing program was set up that turned the lives of many of these troubled adolescents around.

Most of the students had been at other programs and arrived on a load of medication, or they'd been in programs that used M&M's as a reward for good behaviors. So they came in overweight for different reasons and experienced a radical change in diet, with much of the food grown on the farm and a total elimination of sugar drinks, trans fat, and treats. They spent as much time outside as possible and spent up to 65 percent of the day moving. Their sleep was closely monitored and the intrusion of the virtual world limited as much as possible. The treatment worked magic, fairly quickly for some and more gradually for others. Disruptive behaviors diminished, weight dropped, on-task time went way up, and socialization improved.

I am lucky enough to have the chance to re-wild at a health spa at the home of Deborah Szekely. She and her husband created Rancho La Puerta about seventy years ago, and it serves as a re-wilding paradise that people flock to from all over the world. It has exercise at the core, followed by diet—mostly grown on the land here, surrounded by beautiful mountains and flowers, where ever-present bunnies play with the many cats. It is nature in all its glory. Most of the one hundred to two hundred guests spend a large chunk of time sleeping, because there is little to do after dark—no phones, no TV, no Internet except in one small area. You can almost feel the oxytocin flowing while you drop stress by letting yourself down, down, down. There's a three-and-a-half-mile hike up Mount Kuchumaa in the morning, followed by a day chock-full of hourly boot camps, circuit training, African dance, Zumba, yoga, Pilates, tai chi, and more. Here, we are members of a new tribe that sometimes lasts beyond the week.

One of the things that has helped me in my own life is having the ever-present awareness of what happens to my body and mind when I don't incorporate the principles of going wild on a daily basis. I look for ways to fit them in, whether I'm on the road or in the middle of city life in Los Angeles or Boston. I always look for a chance to run or walk outside before my day begins. And after a day with patients in Boston, I jog along the Charles River. When in L.A. with Alicia, I take a ten-minute drive to Franklin Canyon for a hike, surrounded by trees, leaving city life behind, or we head to the infamous Santa Monica Stairs, where the faithful climb up and down a set of stairs while taking in the ocean views. I monitor my sleep much more than before, shutting off the digital world early to try to get enough sleep. I keep taking on new challenges: new playful activities, new projects, new ideas to follow. All of this keeps me mindful just as walking in the woods, sorting through the novel environments, demands that I be present.

RICHARD MANNING

I have been instinctively drawn to wilderness my entire life, so you might think I would have figured out its benefits a long time ago and would not have waited until my sixtieth year to realize the potential of living wild to effect my own well-being. And yet here I am, for the first time in my life, fit, reasonably happy, wholly unmedicated, and optimistic. I weigh less than I did in high school, had to buy all new clothes last year, and run marathon trail races in rocks-and-ice terrain. I am sober. All of this is new.

In truth, this turnaround was a long time coming, a product of a lifetime of thinking and living, and yet the process that led to this book, the thinking and living of these ideas, intensely built a critical mass that can be easily read today in my body and bearing. A long-held tenet of my writing life has been that there is no reason to write a book unless the process of doing so irrevocably changes your life. This book exceeded those expectations.

It's difficult to mark the exact moment, the single thread I pulled to begin unraveling it all, but then it is not altogether arbitrary to say it began in earnest with a fifty-dollar heart monitor. The whole process came together in a flash of realization: I was no longer taking steps to solve a problem. Instead, each new step was directed at exploring how much better life could be. I was no longer salving wounds; I was exploring a potential that seemed limitless.

The heart monitor I owe to John. We met in the summer of 2010, by coincidence, introduced by a mutual friend, Bessel van der Kolk. I read *Spark*, which recommended the heart monitor but also introduced many more important matters. At about the same time, I had admitted to myself that I had become fat and sedentary, and so I would resurrect my long-standing, off-again, on-again relationship with running to get back in shape. I did that but was plagued by injuries and meager results, forcing myself into the daily slog as one would swallow a bitter pill. The heart monitor turned out to be the first step in making the pill less bitter. Inexperienced runners try to run too fast, which is torture while you are doing it but especially in the periods between runs. Too much speed too early makes the activity anaerobic, and this heady level of exertion takes a heavy toll, especially on a fat, old body. I was feeling worse, not better, but a heart monitor slows down those of us who push too hard. It governs a sustained aerobic pace, and then you start to feel better.

I was still fat and depressed, clinically so, but I was moving. Then I happened to read Christopher McDougall's *Born to Run*, and it struck a deep and resonant chord in the wild side of my nature. It said nothing so much as this thing, this running I was somehow driven to do, was driven by evolution. Evolution I knew. What's more, the book argued that I didn't need to pound pavement negotiating a roar of ill-mannered traffic. Running could in fact be done on mountain trails, places I know and love. I live in Montana, and wild is all around, a simple fact that has more to do with my well-being than any other.

But there were deeper tones in the chord. I had long thought and written about environmental well-being, especially about the role of agriculture in reshaping the natural world and our bodies. All of this was summarized in my 2005 book *Against the Grain: How Agriculture Has Hijacked Civilization*. This was more than environmental theory for me. I had adopted a low-carbohydrate diet in the midnineties and have all my life been a hunter. The red meat supply in my house has been dominated by venison and, in Montana, elk and the occasional pronghorn antelope since I was a child. Yet, like John, I was not fanatical about my diet, occasionally lapsing into plates of pasta and, probably much more critically, drinking too much wine and beer.

The ideas about evolution and running in McDougall's book were an exact parallel to the arguments I had long made about food and agriculture: that we were damaging our planet and our lives by ignoring the conditions that shaped us through deep human time. Recognizing that parallel almost instantly, it seems in retrospect, brought me to two thunderbolt realizations: if this was true for food and motion, it must be true for other topics, like sleep and state of mind. But more to the point, if these matters were so fundamental and important to our well-being, they were worth more than intellectual investigation and thought: they were worth living.

Now I play a wild card in the story: neurofeedback, which is becoming an accepted method for treating depression, among other things.

Before I knew depression's proper name, I had my own term, even as a kid: the black hand. I saw it settle periodically on my father, that he would for no reason retreat into brooding silence and anger, it seemed for weeks on end. Soon enough, those habits became my own, and I eventually learned to call this state depression. It is often called "the sadness for no reason," which is

254 • GO WILD

true enough, but it also thrives well if you give it a reason to do so. I had spent a couple of decades leading up to this book writing especially about global environmental degradation, poverty, and government collapse, but not just writing about them. I am a meat-and-potatoes journalist and so researched these matters by traveling and reporting in some of the more desperate corners of the globe.

All of this made me a solid citizen of the Prozac nation, medicated like many for years at a stretch and advised by physicians that these pills would be a condition of the rest of my life. Then I heard about neurofeedback. This technique is a modification of neuroscience's EEG, but it is not simply a passive measure of brain activity. A therapist designates desired areas of the brain and levels of activity that will open up underused neural pathways. The patient watches a display that looks like a video game and that rewards him for using these neural pathways— simple rewards like brighter colors or richer, louder music. No one knows why the patient is able to, almost at will, activate those pathways to achieve the reward, but he does. And because depression, like many other problems, stems from locking into old pathways, using new ones helps make it abate.

I got better, but the technique here is not the point. Plenty of evidence says there are other ways to get a bit better when you have depression, and Prozac is one of them. In retrospect now, though, three years later and unmedicated all that time, I think the real point is how I treated that improvement, not as a cure but as an opportunity, a bit of breathing room, a platform of strength that could be the basis of what else needed to be done.

I have since come to categorize neurofeedback or medication

or tricks like heart monitors and treadmills as essentially the same: they are not solutions. I am not opposed to using them, but they must be used in the right, limited way, the way a builder might use scaffolding as a necessary support to allow the foundation to be built, but then remove it once the project is on more solid ground. If I had stopped with neurofeedback, I would be stuck inhabiting the scaffolding of a life, not a real life.

I began to think very differently about the whole business, and this was the key shift in attitude, the foundation, the core idea that I hope you can take from this book. I abandoned the notion that I was correcting a deficit or fixing a fault. Take the pill and good to go. It occurred to me that I had taken a small step and felt better, so how much "better" was there, how much better could I feel? Were there limits on this? At the outside, what are the limits on human potential for happiness?

July 25, 2011. Unmedicated. Two hundred and ten pounds. A knee sprain has healed to the point of allowing running. This is the day I have chosen to begin, and I quit drinking. I put on a heart monitor. I have selected a marathon, 26.2 miles, and it is five months hence, on New Year's Eve, in Bellingham, Washington, called Last Chance Marathon. Training begins. This is an easy step to plan. Enough people have done this, and enough research has been done that the prescription for a guy in my position—old, fat, and somewhat out of shape—is a matter of consensus. Stay aerobic. Establish a base mileage you can run comfortably and then increase it by no more than 10 percent a week. One long run a week, long and slow. A couple of rest days each week, with no running at all. Maybe a rest week every three weeks or so. There are apps for this. The process is dialed in, and it works pretty well. I finished the marathon. Slow, but finished. I weighed then 185 pounds—25 pounds lighter than when I had begun training five months before.

But what's next? More races out there. I signed up for a thirty-mile trail run, an ultramarathon, in April 2012. I finished, but I was a wreck, crashed into "the wall," not once but at least twice during that run. The wall is that horrible state of fatigue, disorientation, and confusion that strikes distance runners when they have depleted glucose to below the point that the brain needs. The deal was, I was following the standard advice on nutrition, which included heavy doses of carbohydrates and sugar gels administered during long runs. This remains the boilerplate advice of the sport, and I should have known better, understanding well by then the dangers of a high-carb diet. But I figured athletics were the exception, so I took the standard advice. My experience in that first ultra sent me back to the drawing board and resulted in a happenstance change in direction that I now think was my most important discovery.

The reasoning that fronted my doubts about sugar gels and carb-fueled marathons paralleled that found in *Born to Run:* that we'd evolved running without shoes so didn't need them, and in fact probably did damage by running in heavily padded, stiff, heeled shoes. I had taken that advice from the beginning, trained from the start in minimalist "barefoot" shoes, and it had paid off. It allowed me to gear up for ultramarathons without injury. I am a minimalist runner to this day, and it pleases me simply because I have learned that running with unrestricted feet is more fun. No other way to put it. More giggles and smiles in it.

So what about the sugar gels? Hunter-gatherers didn't suck on foil pouches of corn syrup every half hour or so, just as they didn't have foot coffins. Had anyone thought about this? It turns out that people had, especially a guy named Peter Defty and the researchers Steve Phinney and Jeff Volek. They have developed and advocate an ultra-low-carbohydrate school of nutrition called ketogenic, named for the forms of fat that become your fuel. You limit your body to about fifty grams of carbohydrates a day, the total from maybe an apple and turnips at dinner. Fat is your fuel, and in a matter of a couple of weeks, the body adapts. The brain gets the glucose it needs by making it from spare molecular parts, and the metabolic cycle runs on fat. This is probably a reasonable approximation of the way our ancestors ate most of the time, before agriculture. It is of the same order as other low-carbohydrate diets, such as the paleo diet or the Zone, although it's set off from the former by including dairy products. Dairy and lactose are indeed important considerations in finding your particular path, but I seem to have no lactose issues and I like yogurt and cheese, so this is mine.

My goal in this was to run long races without resorting to sucking on sugar water and without crashing with wild undulations of hyper- and hypoglycemia. It worked. Simply and quickly. I can now run as long as seven hours without any food whatsoever, and I never think twice about it. I have since gone for many runs of four hours or more and have never once crashed into a wall. The conventional nutritional wisdom of the sport says this is not supposed to be, but it is, and it's easy.

Almost immediately after changing the way I ate, weight began to fall off my body, although I was not trying to lose weight, nor did I change my running routine, not a bit. I was then and still am running about forty miles a week. But from day one of my ketogenic diet, I began losing about a pound or two a week, step, step, step, in a straight uninterrupted curve until I hit 160 pounds, and then it plateaued and my weight has not varied by more than a pound or two in a year or so since. I pay no attention whatever to total calorie intake, mileage, or the amount of food I eat. Just no sugars. No grains. No processed foods. Lots of nuts, cheese—fat, runny cheeses—bacon, eggs, sausages, sour cream, and vegetables. No high-glycemic fruits like bananas, but apples, pears, and berries, fresh and simple. Lots of venison. Salmon at least once a week. Grass-finished beef. Not a diet. Just the way I eat, and it makes me happy. I repeat, I do not count calories. I am never, ever hungry.

My new eating habits had another unexpected brain benefit, but there is no way I can say for sure that the sum total of my better life stemmed from food choices. Maybe that was just the last piece, the keystone of the arch. Remember, I'd already made the changes with exercise and was at a point in training when I could expect to see some real benefits from running alone. Truly, I had. But remember, too, that this is not about a single intervention; it's more about building a foundation for life.

Still, it was clear that something had worked: my head was getting better. The depression was gone. These changes were no longer an intervention or therapy or cure. They had become my life.

Indeed, I am giving you the barest of outlines of my life during the period, and much that I have left out may in fact be relevant: my solid marriage; the fact that I live in Montana, a wild place; that my work schedule is my own; that I have a dog who runs with me; and that I play music with friends. All of this is relevant, too, and maybe even more so. This is why we can't serve up recipes for others or even research these matters in epidemiological precision. Lives vary, and through time.

OUR PRESCRIPTION FOR YOU

So now it all comes down to the ultimate question: what do you do about all of this? We hope by now it's clear that only you can answer that question fully. But it should also be just as clear that the weight of the evidence offers some sound advice on how one goes about getting better.

First, find your lever. Remember the lever? Beverly Tatum introduced the concept when she told her story about how correcting her sleep deprivation meant she was soon thinking about her nutrition and exercise; the simple act of shutting off her computer at ten each night led to better health on a number of fronts. For Mary Beth Stutzman, the lever was food, specifically carbohydrates. One thing leads to another, and the lever is the key change in your life that triggers others. The first step. Food, microbiome, movement, sleep, mindfulness, tribe, biophilia— all are pieces of the whole.

We don't know what your lever is, but from our own experience, we'd suggest you begin by looking at food or movement or both. We have talked about many issues here, but food and nutrition have been researched the most, are best understood, are profoundly different today from the food and nutrition that formed us as a species, and are so basic to the human condition that it would be hard to imagine anyone getting better without getting these on the right track.

The good news, though, is that it's pretty easy and straightforward to get them on the right track. Here are the basics, and they are simple enough:

Food. Eat no refined sugar in any form. Fructose contained in fresh fruit is okay if not excessive. But no fruit juices. And pay special attention to avoiding sugar dissolved in water: soft drinks but also energy drinks and juices that contain sugar in any form. Don't eat grain. Don't eat anything made from grain. Get your calories from fat, but avoid manufactured fats, otherwise called trans fats. Don't eat processed food. Don't eat fast food. Look for foods high in omega-3 fats, like eggs, grass-finished beef, cold-water fish like salmon, and nuts. Go for simple fresh fruits and vegetables. Go for variety. Eat as much as you like. Enjoy what you eat.

Movement. Look for a form of exercise you like. That comes first. Something you can do easily and as part of your daily routine. Look for forms that involve a variety of movements, full body, with lots of variability, as in both trail running and CrossFit workouts. The gym is okay in a pinch, but look for ways to get outside. Exercise in nature is exercise squared. Feel the sun but also the wind and the rain in your face. Slog through the snow. Get cold. Get hot. Get thirsty. Gear up and go. And especially look for exercise that involves other people. Move with your tribe. Look also to time-honored forms of movement, like dance, qigong, or tai chi. Buy a heart monitor and know your heart. Begin slowly and carefully. Schedule rest days and even rest weeks. And don't stop experimenting and trying new things until you are having fun, until you look forward to each day's run or dance.

If you do these things, you probably will find a lever. Now follow that process as it leads to other steps. Remember, you are no longer checking boxes or putting out fires or whacking moles; you are exploring potential. This process is iterative. Take a step. Assess. Then take another. This whole business becomes not an assignment or duty—rather, an exploration, a process of discovery. It's guided by rewards. So you've been doing this for a couple of weeks. Do you feel better? Want to feel better still? What else is out there? Does the lever lead to better sleep? Awareness? Better engagement with your tribe? Better brain? It should. In time, and not much time, it should.

There is a frustrating irony buried in this whole topic: The more you understand about what needs to be done, the less you are inclined to write about it. Someone once said (the real source is a matter of some debate) that writing about music is a bit like dancing about architecture. The Zen Buddhists have another way of saying pretty much the same thing: meditation is not something you think about; meditation is something you do. Same with well-being. No matter what ails you, you are not going to think your way out of it or read your way out of it. Living well is something you do.

So then it's not something we can do for you as authors, and this realization, too, is informed by our own experience with wilderness. All our lives, we have hiked trails and learned much about life from the experience. Part of the learning comes with finding one's way. This is the lesson of the wild, and to fully realize it, you need to go to the woods and get lost and find your own way, find a trail that suits you.

But we can take you to the trailhead. That's what we have tried to do here, to reveal that there is a series of pathways leading up the mountain and point you to the trailhead. After that, you are on your own.

Acknowledgments

This book was a true collaboration throughout, so the authors accrued common debts to people who helped that process.

We are, of course, grateful to the people we depended on to share information that helped shape and develop our ideas. We identified a number of those when we introduced and quoted them in the text. We have cited key sources and pivotal books. In addition, a number of other people were generous enough with their time and ideas to grant us interviews and give us information and ideas that we used on background but that were still crucial to this work. They include Jennifer Sacheck, a nutritionist at Tufts University; Frank Forencich, who lives in Portland, Oregon, and writes and thinks about the role of movement and play in people's lives; Daniel Lieberman, who is at Harvard and is famous for his ideas on running and evolution; Dennis Bramble, now retired from the University of Utah, who collaborated on a series of pivotal papers with Lieberman; Bryon Powell, editor of the iRunFar website, which covers the world of trail running; Nikki Kimball, a world-class competitive trail runner and a hunter; Martha Herbert, the researcher at Massachusetts

General Hospital known for establishing connections between nutrition and autism; Richard Deth, a researcher in autism at Northeastern University; and Alan Logan, who, with Eva Selhub, wrote *Your Brain on Nature*.

We also got particular help, support, and access from the staff at the Center for Discovery, the forward-looking autism treatment center in New York. We especially thank Terry Hamlin, Matthew Goodwin, and Jenny Foster.

As is the case with most books, this one was borne along to publication by people in the business. Our agent, Peter Matson of Sterling Lord Literistic, served us well in finding a home for these ideas. Tracy Behar, our editor at Little, Brown, was bold enough to take a chance on a big, unruly idea and helped us develop and refine it into what we present here.

In addition to these debts accrued jointly, we also made some severally.

JOHN RATEY

My debt extends to many people who have contributed to my always asking *why* and *why not!* It began as an undergraduate when I was a philosophy major at Colgate and was pushed to think critically of all that I read or thought I knew. It was the late '60s, and exploration of the self and striving for change was the norm. While there, I also lived as a Zen monk for a month and experienced the benefits of meditation, nature, and being in the present.

Then, in medical school at the University of Pittsburgh, I gravitated to some of the best doctors in the land, who seemed to know everything but were secure enough to say they did not. Their honesty was very apparent despite the orthodoxy of medicine. This learned background of uncertainty grew tenfold at the Massachusetts Mental Health Center, were I was guided by my mentors Les Havens, George Vaillant, Richard Shader, and Allan Hobson, who were giants in their fields yet challenged themselves constantly and were never satisfied with the party line. There I began my lifelong association and great friendship with Edward Hallowell, who has been a source of courage and challenge — which has kept me moving toward this end. This determination allowed me to follow the serendipitous leads to develop my work with aggression, then ADHD, and now Go Wild.

This "go for it" attitude to pursue the new or unpopular allowed me to concentrate on the benefits of exercise for the brain. Here I was backed by the science emanating from people such as Carl Cotman, James Blumenthal, Ken Cooper, and Mark Mattson. This eventually led me to what is now a more global appreciation of the brain, mood, and cognition benefits of good living, when most of my tribe were counting on the next drug to come along to push the field forward. I witnessed firsthand the squabbles over the first "scientific" DSM-III, which reinforced the fact that science was unduly influenced by economic and political issues.

I owe much to Phil Lawler and Paul Zientarski, true pioneers who revolutionized their school's physical education program at District 203 in Naperville. In addition, they enlisted me to try to lead their whole profession to change into a more health-and-wellness-oriented discipline. This mission led me to travel the United States, Canada, and around the world to meet many scholars, educators, and movers and shakers who were aware of the problems of the present and wanted to do something about it. The growing awareness that something was not right with our world and the way we were living led me to challenge my own habits.

Finally, I owe a great deal to Richard Manning, a true iconoclast who is a brilliant and tireless intellectual. He is a throwback to the truth-seeking reporter, and our time spent together continues to guide my thinking and sharpen my constructs. Also I am truly grateful to my dear wife, Alicia Ulrich, who continues to share the ideas and ideals we portray in the book.

RICHARD MANNING

My largest debt in any book is usually on the ledger even before I begin, with the help I get leading up to the genesis of an idea. This one is no exception, and goes way back to the 1980s, when I read a profile of Wes Jackson in *Atlantic* magazine. Jackson, the great agronomist and MacArthur genius, had the idea of reinventing agriculture to make it wild, "farming in nature's image," he called it. This revolutionary notion led me to years of thinking about wildness, food, and the essence of who we are.

In recent years, though, I have been oddly steered through the last of those—human essence—through a chance encounter with Rick van den Pol, who runs the Institute for Educational Research and Service at the University of Montana. My work with Rick soon steered me to the seminal ideas of Bessel van der Kolk and then a chance meeting with John Ratey, van der Kolk's good friend. I am indebted to all of these people, but especially to John, whose vast knowledge of the human brain and groundbreaking ideas on the importance of exercise and movement helped close the circle almost thirty years in the making. Throughout this process, he was inspirational and thoroughly patient with my meanderings and quixotic tendencies, not to mention he deftly corrected some of my more boneheaded and embarrassing errors of fact. He was broad-minded enough to partner with an unrepentant journalist, an ink-stained wretch, and I thank him for it.

My other major debt piled up during every day of the writing of this book and is really owed to a place, not some people—or, more to the point, to the people who preserve the place. During part—the most important part—of almost every day for the months of writing, I ran on a remarkable series of mountain trails that weaves the rim of the valley that holds Helena, Montana. This setting was crucial to the writing process, provided some scenes that appear in this book, and anchored the project in the wilds of the Northern Rockies. During a week John and I spent hammering through the edits on a first draft, we both hit these same trails every day together. The debt here accrues to the Prickly Pear Land Trust, a nonprofit in Helena that has taken it upon itself to acquire the land and easements and do the literal pick-and-shovel work that allows this system to exist and, in the process, makes Helena a biophilic city. Bless them.

This, however, is only a short chunk of trail compared to the long, twisted, and far more treacherous path stretching back to the point where I met a young woman named Tracy Stone, now my wife. Only she knows the full difficulty of the terrain leading to this point, because she has been with me every step of the way, and I couldn't have done it without her. The true paradox here is that all of my other debts are trivial in comparison, yet this one is the easiest to bear.

Index

About the Authors

JOHN J. RATEY, MD, is a clinical associate professor of psychiatry at Harvard Medical School. He is the author or coauthor of numerous bestselling and groundbreaking books, including *Spark, Driven to Distraction,* and *A User's Guide to the Brain.* He lives in Cambridge, Massachusetts, and Los Angeles.

RICHARD MANNING is an award-winning journalist. He is the author of nine books, including *Against the Grain* and *One Round River.* His work has appeared in *The Best American Science and Nature Writing 2010, Harper's,* the *New York Times,* the *Los Angeles Times,* and other publications. He lives in Helena, Montana.